THROUGH,

NOT

AROUND

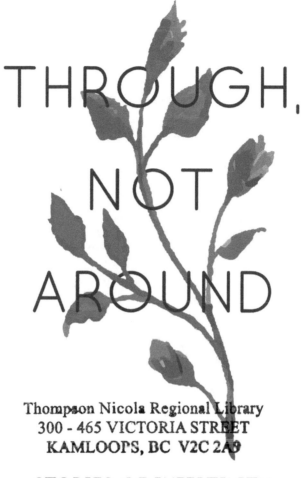

THROUGH, NOT AROUND

STORIES OF INFERTILITY AND PREGNANCY LOSS

ALLISON McDONALD ACE
ARIEL NG BOURBONNAIS
CAROLINE STARR

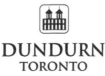

DUNDURN
TORONTO

Cover image: Creative Market | Olga Alekseenko
Printer: Webcom, a division of Marquis Book Printing Inc.

Library and Archives Canada Cataloguing in Publication

Through, not around : stories of infertility and pregnancy loss / edited by Allison McDonald Ace, Caroline Starr, Ariel Ng Bourbonnais.

Issued in print and electronic formats.
ISBN 978-1-4597-4296-3 (softcover).--ISBN 978-1-4597-4297-0 (PDF).--
ISBN 978-1-4597-4298-7 (EPUB)

1. Miscarriage--Psychological aspects. 2. Infertility—Psychological aspects. 3. Pregnancy--Psychological aspects. 4. Grief. I. McDonald Ace, Allison, editor II. Starr, Caroline, editor III. Ng Bourbonnais, Ariel, editor

RG648.T57 2019   362.1966'92   C2018-905374-7
                                              C2018-905375-5

1 2 3 4 5   23 22 21 20 19

 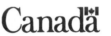

We acknowledge the support of the **Canada Council for the Arts**, which last year invested $153 million to bring the arts to Canadians throughout the country, and the **Ontario Arts Council** for our publishing program. We also acknowledge the financial support of the Government of Ontario, through the **Ontario Book Publishing Tax Credit** and **Ontario Creates**, and the **Government of Canada**.

Nous remercions le **Conseil des arts du Canada** de son soutien. L'an dernier, le Conseil a investi 153 millions de dollars pour mettre de l'art dans la vie des Canadiennes et des Canadiens de tout le pays.

Care has been taken to trace the ownership of copyright material used in this book. The author and the publisher welcome any information enabling them to rectify any references or credits in subsequent editions.
— *J. Kirk Howard, President*

The publisher is not responsible for websites or their content unless they are owned by the publisher.

Printed and bound in Canada.

VISIT US AT

 dundurn.com | 🐦 @dundurnpress | 📘 dundurnpress | 📷 dundurnpress

Dundurn
3 Church Street, Suite 500
Toronto, Ontario, Canada
M5E 1M2

To the ones who came before us and the ones who will come after

CONTENTS

INTRODUCTION

AS WITH MOST THINGS, this book came to be through a series of events that none of us had planned and, if we had the chance, we all would change. No one has the luxury of choice when it comes to joining the Pregnancy Loss and Infertility Club. While everything doesn't always happen for a reason — tragedy is sometimes just that, tragedy — it is abundantly clear from the thread woven through each story told by our brave authors in this collection that out of tragedy can come the greatest of gifts: gratitude, compassion, empathy, hope, patience, humour, and, most importantly, the resilience to go on living and loving when everything inside of you wants to give up.

This kind of resilience and strength doesn't show up in the loud, bombastic way we've come to expect from movies. This kind of resilience lives in the quietest and innermost places of those who embody it the most, and it's only when they allow us a window into that inner world that we are able to see just what they are made of. And as you will see from the view we've provided here, those of us who've unwillingly joined this club are made of strong stuff.

As co-editors and co-authors of this book, we all felt an immense responsibility to give voice to as many facets of the experience of pregnancy loss and infertility as possible so that our readers may find within these pages the knowledge that they — or you — are not alone. Because, truly, you are not. You might also find comfort in knowing that it could be worse. No one ever wants to admit to these thoughts, but if in reading this book you find that you can go on because your battle is less arduous than someone else's, we are here to give you permission to feel that way. These stories are being told to help you go on moving forward, in whatever way you can.

We launched The 16 Percent, an online community that shares stories of loss and infertility that eventually gave birth (pun intended) to this book. We wanted to create that space because we knew, viscerally, from our own experiences, that telling our stories is the way through the grief and a way to cope. Most importantly, to declare out loud that you are sad, enraged, terrified, and confused is to declare that it is okay to feel this way and that it is not your job to carry this burden quietly so those around you may be comfortable. Your story matters. Your experience is unique. Your voice should be heard if you want to share your story to help others heal. The more we tell these stories and give voice to what it's like to lose a child or be unable to carry one into this world, the more we allow this part of life and the act of sharing to be a little less scary for those who come after us on this path.

Speaking of which, this path is not one that comes with a map. When we each found ourselves suddenly and unexpectedly staring down this unfamiliar road, we had to figure out how to navigate that bumpy terrain as best as possible without a guide. But it is our hope that within the hard-won knowledge of these stories, we are now able to offer a map to guide you. You will find that there is no way to the other end of the path but to follow it to the end. You can try to pick a different route or take a short cut around the path, but ultimately you will find yourself back on it. And the reason for this is that the path is there for you: not to hurt you, but to lead you out — out of grief, out of being stuck, and, eventually, to where your life is waiting. It may not be the life you planned, but it is yours and it wants you to live it. So, if ever you're feeling lost, please hold fast to the directions we give you here. They are simple to remember, although not always easy to follow:

The way forward is through, not around.

In the following essays, some names and identifying details have been changed to protect the privacy of individuals.

1

HOW TO BE (INFERTILE) IN THE WORLD

Wendy Litner

I'M ON MY WAY TO an infertility support group and I hate what I'm wearing: jeans and a button-down shirt. I should have worn that vintage pink dress that makes me feel like Baby the night of the big show. This isn't the kind of infertile I wanted to look like. I have been feeling this way a lot lately. I cut my hair, shorter than I usually do, and I like it, but still it isn't enough. I wish I could unzip my skin, opening a seam from the top of my head to the backs of my heels, and step right out of myself. Everything about me just feels wrong from the outside in. Or maybe it's the inside out? I don't know anymore.

I survey the other women every morning at the fertility clinic, take note of their shoes, their purses, their tops, and their skirts, and despite the fact that we are all battling the same thing, they all seem right in a way that I am wrong. They are coping with infertility far more stylishly than I am, and it makes me terribly sad because I want to have a baby but I also want to be dressed right. I imagine they are all wearing lovely lacy underwear, too, which they fold neatly on the chair beside them as they get undressed for their exam. Mine are cotton.

When our ultrasound numbers are called, we form a single line behind the technician, who asks each of us, every morning, one after another, if we've "gone to the washroom." It feels odd every time to be asked out loud, as a grown woman, if you've recently peed. It always seems more incongruous to ask this question of a woman in heels. I'm embarrassed for the ones in heels especially. But we are asked all the same, I in my ballet flats or sometimes my slip-on Chucks, and they in their impressive pumps. *Do these women really have transvaginal ultrasounds and then put their heels back on?* I wonder. I'm impressed by their sartorial stamina.

I took a week-long writing course at the Humber School for Writers a few years back, and when I was frustrated, struggling to knit pieces of my story together into something cohesive, my teacher, Bruce Jay Friedman, said to me, "If it ain't rough, it ain't right." *Yes*, I thought, *Yes!* The process of creating something *should be* difficult and uneasy and altogether rough! I asked Bruce to write this quote, said by former Detroit Piston Chauncey Billups, on a page of my notebook. He did, and I've kept it among other torn pages of notebooks for some future reference. I planned to tape the quote over my desk for inspiration, to remind me that important things are usually hard and take work. I think about it now, though, realizing it doesn't actually mean anything. Not really. When things are good and truly rough, pithy little sayings don't really mean anything at all. Because you could be more right, couldn't you? You could wear Ferragamo shoes (those ones with the bow) and non–American Eagle brand jeans. And you could get pregnant on your own, like you're supposed to. Like all your friends have. Like all your family has.

I should have worn the pink Baby dress.

There is a man with a guitar singing "Take It Easy" as I wait for the subway to pull into the station, and I have the urge to yell at him, "No, *you*! *You* take it easy." I then fear I am becoming bitter and wonder if this is what becomes of the childless. They get angry at harmless buskers with moderately good voices singing the Eagles on subway platforms. I think this often, substituting whatever my bad behaviour is that day and wonder if it's a hallmark of people who want children and can't have them. *So this is what becomes of the childless. They are put off by people in coffee shops who sit beside them and cough emphatically without covering their mouths?*

I watch a mother take her son and start slow dancing to the music. The boy looks to be about eight, so at first he's embarrassed, but then she dips him and he laughs like, "Oh, Mom," like this is just so endearingly her, and I say to myself, *I hope I'm that kind of mom, the kind that dances to shitty subway music while waiting for the train to come.* I'm always plotting out the kind of mother I want to be. I have a folder in my Gmail where I save articles on how to get a baby to sleep, how to settle a toddler having a tantrum in the middle of a grocery store, how to talk to children about race. I like the advice they have to give, and I email the articles to myself because I don't know what else to do. I want to be a really good mother to the little boy or the little girl I can't get pregnant with. I can't have him or her throwing hissy fits in grocery stores and be totally unprepared.

I usually make it a personal policy not to participate in anything that requires a name tag, but I fear I have exhausted my family and friends with the incessant discussion about the state of my fertility. I thought a support group would remind me that I am not the only woman in the world who can't get pregnant, despite all the lovely women I see on a daily basis pushing strollers past me, doing whatever it is people who can have babies do.

The women here already seem to know each other's names. The group meets the second-last Thursday of every month and there are clearly regulars. I thought I would find here what writer Pamela Mahoney Tsigdinos calls a "silent sorority," where we envelop each other in our commiseration and say things like, "Ass Injections, amiright?"

Infertility has few awareness walks and no coloured ribbons, yet it still has its own sad subculture of people who must remember far too many acronyms. Having difficulty conceiving is all the rage right now, with Elizabeth Banks discussing how her baby was born via surrogate, Nicole Kidman sharing details of her miscarriages, and Chrissy Teigen tweeting about conceiving via in vitro fertilization, or IVF (if I could look like any kind of infertile, it would be her).

I'm both overwhelmed by my infertility and fear its absorption. I recall flipping through the book *How to Be Parisian Wherever You Are,* an enduring goal of mine, though I have lost my ability to speak French, and it said, "The word 'pregnant' is an adjective. It describes you, it doesn't define you." I feel the same, then, must be true of the word *infertile.*

So what am I doing here? Taking comfort in my infertility while not being defined by it, I suppose. It's a fine line, when you attend a fertility clinic morning after morning for blood tests and transvaginal ultrasounds and get daily injections in the ass and stomach, layered on top of other medication all designed to have you grow eggs, which will hopefully grow into a baby, who will change your life forever.

We sit in a circle in the waiting room of the clinic, and I wonder if we will go around and say our names and declare our infertility: "Hello. My name is Wendy and I've been infertile now for two and half years." The moderator begins with some introductory thoughts on infertility and how this is a safe space to discuss our feelings. I feel a rising wave of panic as she speaks. I look around and study the faces of the other women. They all look like versions of me: 30-something, tired and frustrated and confused and sad. I want to take comfort in our mutually sad experience, but I also want to back away, my arms covering my face, and say, "No, no, I am nothing like you!" Because fertility treatments might fail them, but they are eventually going to work for me, aren't they? This latest cycle I am in the middle of is going to work. Isn't it? It has to. It must. I've read the statistics now about the success rates for IVF and, looking around the circle, I'm acutely aware that some of us are going to be on the wrong side of the numbers. But not me. It can't be me.

The moderator's words fall at my feet as I'm busy appraising each woman, wondering who among us will be the first out of the group to get pregnant. I wonder if they are all playing the same game, and I hope so much they think it's me. I want it to be me, to never have reason to come back here again. But it's not me; it's the woman sitting beside me.

"I'm pregnant!" she announces. There is a chorus of limp congratulations. She tells us how the doctor, whose waiting room we are meeting in tonight, said she would definitely need assisted reproductive technology to have a second child, a notion she rejected in favour of meditation and fertility yoga. So there she went, rejecting medical intervention, meditating, and yoga-ing, and now she's pregnant. She's fucking pregnant.

The moderator says we are allowed to feel a little stung by this news — but not really, because this woman has been coming to group for a while now, and even though she already gets to be a mother, it took her a long time to get pregnant the second time. So it's okay. It's okay that she didn't need to subject herself to the torture of fertility treatments. It's okay that she miraculously got pregnant on her own and came to share the news at an infertility support group. She's come, she says, "to give the rest of us hope!" Oh, and incidentally, she has started an infertility yoga practice if any of us would like her business card. I decline (but I search Google for fertility yoga the moment I get home).

The conversation naturally moves on to the benefits of meditation and yoga and acupuncture, and the conclusion is that these things can't really hurt; they can only help.

I clear my throat. "I'm having a really hard time knowing just what to do with myself," I say. "Every single decision feels weighty and suspect. I want to try yoga to relax myself, but then I'm scared of bending and twisting and damaging my few growing eggs. I tried acupuncture but it made me nauseated, and then I worried about taking Gravol. This woman I know sent me an email warning me about a link between infertility and eating GMO foods, which I thought was crazy, but then I found myself spending a mortgage payment on fucking kale and kale-related products at the organic grocery store. I rest because I am so tired from all the medication, and then jog around the block because I'm worried about blood flow to my uterus, and then I don't know what to do with myself, so I strike fucking warrior pose just to do something, anything. I don't know how to live anymore! I don't know what to do with myself anymore! I want to be a mother so badly I don't know how to be in the world anymore!"

My voice cracks and I'm breathless, my chest heaving with all my pent-up frustrations at having to live as if I'm pregnant even though I'm not. I feel panicked and sorry for swearing in front of the conservative-looking woman sitting beside me. I blink back my tears.

The women look at each other in silence. Then, finally, the moderator nods her head.

"It can all be very confusing, can't it?" she says.

And then someone asks about taking Coenzyme Q10 and whether it can really rejuvenate your eggs by 10 years. I've been taking it myself for almost a year and still have the shitty eggs of a 35-year-old. I don't say this, though, to the woman who asked about it, because she looks so very hopeful and at least 40 and she has no children, so I agree with everyone, that, yes, Coenzyme Q10 can't really hurt; it can only help.

The group ends with each of us saying something we hope to do over the next month: try a new restaurant, go back to the gym. "Have a baby," I joke, when it's my turn. No one laughs. As I grab my coat and purse to leave, peel off my name tag from the shirt I don't like, a woman approaches me.

"I appreciate what you said," she says.

I apologize for saying "fuck" so much.

She laughs.

I like her. I hope this works for her. I hope she gets pregnant.

2

AGAINST MIRACLES

Teri Vlassopoulos

IT'S DIFFICULT DECIDING where to begin and then where to draw the line with fertility treatments. At the beginning, you tell yourself that if it doesn't happen, it doesn't happen. You imagine your life without a baby and all the travelling you and your husband will do together, how many books you'll write. But as roadblocks litter your path, you hedge your initial position: if it doesn't happen, it doesn't happen, sure, but why not try this first before giving up? And … this. And this, too.

You get accustomed to treatments and acclimatize yourself step by step. You grapple with questions of how comfortable you are with what you're getting yourself into. While you wouldn't balk at medical interventions to save a life, it's another thing to rely on them to create a new one.

And as much as you hoped you could be casual about it, as much as you wish you could think through your decisions rationally, you can't. There is fate, but there are also things you can do to massage your life into the future you want. Coax it in the right direction.

You are often exhausted without being able to pinpoint exactly why.

My story isn't unique. My husband, Andrew, and I tried for a baby; nothing happened. After six months, I brought it up with my doctor. "Just in case,"

I tried to say breezily, as if I weren't really concerned. She scheduled tests for both of us, and as a result of Andrew's sperm analysis, we jumped into intrauterine insemination (IUI) right away.

While problems are relatively simple to diagnose on the male side, they're more opaque when it comes to women. It wasn't uncommon for us to think we had a handle on our problems, only to get a call from a nurse with a prescription for a drug for me to take to regulate a hormonal issue that, a month earlier, I had no idea existed. So when multiple rounds of IUI failed and another half year had passed, our next step was in vitro fertilization (IVF).

In retrospect, it sounds methodical, like we were following a flowchart, but at the time it felt as though we were inching our way through a dark, twisty maze. I wasn't sure where we'd end up or how long it would take for me to get pregnant or if I would get pregnant at all.

After our first IVF consultation, we came home with a thick folder of information. I wanted to know all the details but I was intimidated, so I paged through the materials quickly until the description of the embryo transfer slowed me down.

During the transfer, the five-day-old blastocyst embryo is microscopic: less than 0.2 millimetres in diameter. It's loaded into a catheter, which is inserted into the uterus, and then squeezed out, where it will hopefully implant. I'd assumed the process of IVF was sturdy with science, but learning the exact measurements of the embryo made me realize we were creating something impossibly small, the size of the period at the end of this sentence. How would it not get crushed during all that human, error-prone handling? If someone accidentally sneezed, it might shatter. To be paying thousands of dollars for this seemed in vain, but we'd already gone so far down this path, and besides, what else could we do?

The Brothers Grimm's *The Sleeping Beauty* starts off with this: "In times past there lived a King and Queen, who said to each other every day of their lives, 'Would that we had a child!' and yet they had none." It's not until the queen is visited by a frog who prophesizes a daughter that they're finally graced with one.

Hans Christian Andersen's *Thumbelina* begins similarly: "There once was a woman who wanted so very much to have a tiny little child, but she did not know where to find one. So she went to an old witch, and she said: 'I have set my heart upon having a tiny little child. Please, could you tell me where I can find one?'" The answer, it turned out, was a grain of barley that when planted produced a strange flower that unfurled itself to reveal a literal tiny little child.

That's what I'd expected from the clinic: prophetic frogs and magic barley grains. Instead, what we were given was cruder, more sterile. Synthetic hormones injected from a syringe. The snowy gradient of an ultrasound screen. Soft catheter tubing, a swab, a petri dish. I wanted more. Something like a fairy tale; something more miraculous.

This word *miracle*, defined by Oxford Dictionaries as "an extraordinary and welcome event that is not explicable by natural or scientific laws and is therefore attributed to a divine agency," is used often when it comes to babies. Most frequently, it's used to explain the ordinary phenomenon of getting pregnant. For a word reserved for something extraordinary, it's thrown around casually.

"During the early months you may become more introspective as you consider the miracle going on inside you," Dr. Sears advises mothers in the first section of *The Healthy Pregnancy Book*. Yet in the past five years, Canadians have on average given birth to 386,000 babies per year, more than 1,000 each day. That's a lot of miracles.

Miracle is also used frequently in the world of infertility. The first babies born in North America from IVF lived in Oakville, just outside of Toronto. It was 1982 — four years after the first successful IVF — and their parents had travelled to the United Kingdom to work directly with the doctors who had pioneered the fertility treatment. They returned to Canada to give birth to twin boys, made newspaper headlines, and then went on with their lives. When one of the twins eventually became a father, a handful of articles popped up. His baby, a perfectly average 7-pound-12-ounce boy, and the conception, achieved the old-fashioned way, were not particularly notable, but since the father's birth had been part of a new narrative arc, the birth of his own child tied a neat bow on the circle of life. The father demurred though. "Every birth is a bit of a miracle," he told the *London*

Free Press. But if a regular pregnancy is a miracle, then one that happens against all odds must be even *more* miraculous.

And, at its heart, this is the problem with being accustomed to the vocabulary of miracles when it comes to childbearing: it ends up equating failure of conception or birth with a divine curse. If you're trying, but not having a baby, there isn't just something biologically wrong with you; there's also something cosmically, spiritually wrong.

Maybe this is why I was so tired.

When our first IVF attempt failed, I knew I needed distractions. Andrew and I took a trip to New York City and revelled in travelling with no responsibilities, not concerned about whether or not we should drink, not having to rush to the clinic by 6:30 every morning so that we weren't late for work. Going through infertility had made our relationship stronger — the way Andrew was able to make me laugh when I felt my worst or how he would come with me to an appointment without hesitation for moral support even if he wasn't required reaffirmed this — but it was hard to focus on the more lighthearted parts of our relationship when our lives revolved so tightly around fertility treatments.

Finally, I signed up for pottery classes. I said it was because I'd always wanted to learn, but deep down I knew it was more because if I couldn't make a baby, I could at least make something else while I waited. I was also sick of being stuck inside my head, of worrying, of imagining all the worst possible scenarios. Pottery classes, then, would be perfect. For three hours a week, my mind would have a break from those thoughts as I worked with my hands. Even better, I would have tangible proof of my efforts.

I secretly thought I would be good at pottery. I had vague memories of easily moulding shapes out of Play-Doh as a child. Despite my reproductive difficulties, I'd forgotten that the simplest things are often the hardest to make. A bowl, a plate. Shapes you should be able to make from muscle memory, but when you try to replicate them, you realize you were never taught how to do so in the first place.

At the first class, the teacher showed our small group how to pinch off some clay and knead it until it was pliable. Once it was ready for the wheel, it was time to centre. You take your lump of clay and smack it down in the middle of the wheel. You then cup it between your wet hands, and as the wheel spins you form the lump into a dome. If you don't centre the clay properly, it will show in your finished project. Your pots will be off-kilter; they will warp, or worse, collapse into a wet pile of clay so you'll be forced to start over again from scratch. Our teacher demonstrated a few times and then made us try.

"I did it," I said, proud of myself for mastering the skill so quickly. Our teacher could eyeball a wheel from across a room and tell if the clay on it was wobbly.

"Great try," she said. She came over and fixed it with a quick sleight of hand. "See?"

It seemed so simple when she centred the clay, but as much as I tried, I could never do it myself. *I'll figure it out by the third class*, I thought. *No, the fourth.* But it wasn't intuitive to me, and whenever a bowl went wonky, it could be traced back to my failure to centre the clay. Often I would try my best and then ask my teacher to tweak it so I could just move on to the next step.

When my bowls and cups were glazed and fired, I loved them, imperfections and all. But a part of me was sheepish that I hadn't fully centred them myself, that they were all made with a little help. Was it cheating? Did I really need help for *everything*, from baby-making to now this, what was supposed to be a lighthearted hobby, a distraction? Did it matter? They were mostly my creations. I just needed a boost at the very beginning.

Months passed. Another IVF cycle didn't work; I signed up for another session of pottery classes. We had a frozen-embryo transfer scheduled, but I was wary. Initially, it had been comforting knowing that it was possible to bank embryos. It meant that the physical lengths I had gone to during the egg retrieval wouldn't go to waste. But I also found it hard to believe that an embryo could not only survive a deep freeze, but then go on to flourish. Humans were not designed to thrive in sustained cold; other mammals can hibernate in the winter, but we can't. Our systems don't allow it.

As the date approached, I revisited our informational packet. Our clinic used a freezing technique discovered in the early 2000s called embryo vitrification. Unlike the old method, vitrification is practically instantaneous, a freeze so quick that ice crystals that might corrupt the embryo's cells don't get the chance to form. The word for the process is unusually poetic, too, especially in comparison to the scientific lexicon of fertility treatments. *Vitrine*, a glass cabinet to store your precious things, your fine bone china, your Fabergé eggs. I imagined a Christmas display of shimmering glass ornaments, or a window on a winter day, the pattern of crystallized ice against the glass intricate and beautiful. The informal term for a child born from a frozen embryo is *snow baby*, one of those overly cutesy phrases you'll see on infertility message boards, embarrassing until you fall for it, too, as you picture a ruddy-cheeked baby swaddled in soft furs, nestled in a snowdrift. You have been walking through a storm for days, for months, for years, and then you look down. *Oh, there you are! Come, let me warm you up.*

The day before the transfer, Andrew and I went to the Art Gallery of Ontario to see a new Henry Moore retrospective. We needed the distraction. I'd always admired Moore's work and the way he scored and etched plaster casts to look like worn-down bone. At the gallery, I stopped in front of one of his larger works, *Woman*, a giant seated nude of a woman with huge breasts and hips and then, up top, a tiny pin of a head. Many of Moore's sculptures focus on the female form, but this one, I read, was specifically a tribute to fertility. "The smallness of the head is necessary to emphasize the massiveness of the body," he'd written about her. "If the head had been any larger, it would have ruined the whole idea of the sculpture."

Standing there, I felt like the complete opposite of *Woman*. That the head wasn't an important part of his representation of fertility bothered me. If I'd made the sculpture myself, the head would've been huge, swollen with thoughts and worries and hopes. It was as important as those hips, those breasts. I was suddenly furious. *Fuck you, Henry Moore*, I thought. *I will prove you wrong.*

A few days after our transfer, I became aware of my breasts in a way I hadn't been before. *It's probably nothing*, I told myself, but they felt like a bigger part of me, emphasized, almost grudgingly, like *Woman*'s. The feeling didn't go away, and two weeks later I woke up early to take a pregnancy test. Andrew was still in bed, and when he heard me gasping as I walked back to the bedroom clutching the stick, he assumed the worst. I sat down next to him and showed him what the test had indicated almost immediately after I'd peed on it. Two lines.

And then I was pregnant. The miracle was not so much that it had happened, but that the time waiting to get to that point — just over two years — suddenly softened, stopped feeling like such a tax, a burden. In the same way that the pain of childbirth loses its intensity after the baby is born, the sharpness of infertility shifted from a sting to a duller throb. The pain didn't go away, but it became easier to ignore.

I had taken note of another Moore sculpture that day in the gallery. *Mother and Child* was inspired by Moore's wife nursing his daughter. Unlike his other motherhood sculptures, all rounded corners and soft curves, this one is almost violent. The baby's face is bird-like, its sharp beak lunging for its mother's breast. The mother, her head with a serrated edge to it, clutches the strange creature tightly. Informally, Moore called the sculpture "Nora" because when he saw his daughter at his wife's breast, he thought it looked like she was gnawing her. "Gnaw her" = "Nora." Unlike *Woman*, this sculpture didn't anger me. I suspected there was maybe a kind of truth to it.

In the early days after our baby was born, I sometimes thought of *Mother and Child*. Usually it would be in the middle of the night, when we were all be in bed together in a sleepy twilight haze. The way my daughter lunged toward my breast, ferocious even though her eyes were closed, was enough to remind me that we were animals. Our behaviour was pure animal instinct: her feeding, my feelings of protectiveness, the surge of overwhelming love. It was all natural, despite the lengths we took to get there, despite the hours spent in the sterile environment of a clinic downtown.

I eventually looked into why Moore was so obsessed with fertility and motherhood. I'd assumed it was because he was awash in these images, that his life had a fecundity to it that naturally spilled over into his work. But that turned out not to be the case: Moore had one daughter, Mary, who was born when he was 47. His wife, Irina, was 39, and she had a series of miscarriages before Mary arrived. While Moore had already made some female-form sculptures, it was Mary's birth that marked the increase.

I realized that this made more sense than my original assumption. Obsessions are rarely steeped in what we have in abundance; they're based on things we want but can't have, or that we had and then lost, or what we finally manage to get, but only barely, by the skin of our teeth.

So what was the right formula for making a baby? Was it waiting for some-one divine outside ourselves to say, "It is now your turn; you are blessed"? Was it something complicated and subtle, like turning a wet lump of clay into a smooth, sturdy vessel? Was it the sum product of x number of early morning clinic appointments and y vials of medication? Even after I had given birth, the question weighed on my mind. I had been desperate for a clear path, even in hindsight, and I wanted to summarize it with the simple elegance of a fairy tale.

Eventually I came across Frida Kahlo's painting, *Henry Ford Hospital*. Kahlo never had children but had many miscarriages, and the painting was an explicit representation of one of her experiences that occurred when she accompanied Diego Rivera to Detroit, where he'd been commissioned to paint frescoes at the Detroit Institute of Arts. In the painting, Kahlo is cry-ing, curled up naked on a hospital bed with blood blooming on the white sheets. She holds six strings, each tied to a different object hovering around her like a balloon: a fetus, a grey snail, an anatomical model of a female abdomen, a stainless steel machine, an orchid, and a pelvis. They represent different parts of the miscarriage — it wasn't just about the fetus, but also the slowness of the situation, the medical intervention, the impacts on her body, and finally, a glimmer of beauty.

While the painting depicted a miscarriage, I could easily relate it to my experience with infertility. The assortment of objects was a more accurate way to describe what goes into conceiving a child when you can't simply rely on divine order.

Ultimately, the things that helped me understand the complexity of what I felt, of what had happened, were completely unrelated to the actual mechanics of reproduction: pottery, sculptures, a painting. Something as simple as a fairy tale never could have captured it all. But my favourite stories were never fairy tales anyway. I've always preferred the circuitous ones, the ones with plot twists, minor characters, and surprise endings where happiness isn't a guarantee, but a privilege. And so, despite acknowledging that good fortune had a part in the conception of our daughter, I don't think I can say it was a miracle. It was more than that.

3

A QUIET FUNERAL

Allison McDonald Ace

WE STAND AWKWARDLY in the cold, sunny February afternoon, me holding what's left of my baby in a burgundy velvet pouch that fits into the palm of my hand. My mom is holding a potted white daisy she picked up because it was the only thing available at the store. We all know it will die in the cold, but it feels wrong to just put her in the ground without anything to mark her place. So we all pretend like it will last.

My baby has no name because I'm still holding on to the name, reserving it. I'm hoping for a chance to give it to a live baby, not a dead one. And because her heart stopped beating three days before the 20-week mark, we aren't required by the law to give her a "real" burial. This is a relief to me, because I don't want to be someone who's had a funeral for her baby, even one that I only carried in my body, even one who never even took a breath of air. Somehow that would make this story more tragic, and it's tragic enough for me.

We are burying her remains in the garden bed of my family's plot in a cemetery, surrounded by the graves of mostly Chinese families who've placed elaborate offerings of food and candles and incense for their lost ones. Our daisy that will not last the week suddenly seems even more pathetic.

My husband stands a foot behind my mom and me, taking up his own space to grieve. My dad sits on the bench with my grandfather's last name etched into it, with a look on his face that is a mix of sadness and restlessness. I'm pretty sure he's wondering how long this makeshift funeral is actually going to take. Not because he doesn't care — but, rather, because he cares too much and can sit only so long in the pain and the sadness of what we are doing.

None of us has ever been to a makeshift funeral, let alone been the orchestrators of one. The last time we stood at this gravesite was to bury Papa, and Granny a few years before him. Both burials came with all the pomp and circumstance befitting one who has lived a full and complete life. But my baby never had a full life, not even half a life, or a day of real, outside-my-body life, and so this feels more fitting to me somehow, to be making up the rules as we go along to fit the circumstances. I'm conscious of not being overly dramatic about the whole thing because I don't want to make more of this than it needs to be. I'm not sure who I'm worried about more: me or my parents or my husband. I only know that if I don't give in to this too much, if I hold a little back, then somehow we will all be protected by that.

For a while we just stand in silence, the deceptively warm sunshine beating down on us to keep the cold winter air at bay. Probably for the 27th time this week, I feel relieved that at the last minute I called the hospital to say that, in fact, I did want the funeral home to collect my baby's remains for cremation. My husband and I had originally decided at the hospital, after they surgically removed my daughter from my body, that she could just stay there, with them. That because we didn't have to give her a burial, we wouldn't. As if that would help us to forget sooner or heal faster. But as the days went on back at home and I lay on the couch, unable to move, thinking and crying, crying and thinking, the idea of allowing her tiny body to be disposed of as medical waste was not something I could live with. The idea that I almost let that happen makes me want to vomit. But there are no rules to follow when your baby dies just shy of 20 weeks. Because she's not considered an actual human.

And yet, because I was five months pregnant, she was too big for me to undergo a dilation and curettage (D&C) to suction her out of me, so I was told that I would have to be induced and deliver her vaginally, just like with any other baby. This was said to me in a casual way, as if of course I would have to push a dead baby out of my body. As I tried to wrap my head around the fact that my first vaginal birth — my son had been born via emergency Caesarean section — would be for a not-live baby, the nurses also dropped in the fact that I'd suddenly developed a complete placenta previa sometime between my last ultrasound and that day. And because of that I would have to push the placenta out first. It would have to break into a dozen small pieces to even allow for my baby to leave my body, which would likely result in huge blood loss requiring potential blood transfusions.

No big deal.

Whether because of real instinct or raw, primal fear I'll never know, but in that moment I felt in my bones that if I went along with their plan, I was most certainly going to die. The notion that I would possibly be leaving my living son behind spurred me to insist, argue, and advocate for my instincts with the conviction of a mother bear, even though I had barely enough energy left to account for a small mouse. Thanks to my obstetrician, who actually gives a shit about what her patients have to say, I won over the powers that be and they all agreed to a change in plans. I would instead undergo a hysterotomy, which is basically a Caesarean section but with a smaller, vertical incision, because my baby didn't require that much room for manoeuvring. They also decided that I didn't need to be awake for the procedure, since that was reserved for people who wanted to see their babies being pulled out, to hear their babies' cries, and to hold their babies in their arms.

I never saw my baby. I never held her in my arms. Maybe it was self-preservation, but I was worried the image of holding my not-live baby would haunt me more than anything else, and so in my detached state I also figured I didn't need to bury her, that I could just put the entire experience in a small compartment that didn't require more than a surgery to move on from. But as we stand in the cemetery, I am comforted knowing she is going to be with my family in this place, surrounded by their spirits and their names carved in stone. And also the Chinese ancestors, for good measure.

Breaking me out of my daze, my mom hands me a small shovel she brought from home, which I recall being forced to use over so many summers to help her plant impatiens even though I hated gardening. I bend down and dig a tiny hole, just like she taught me to do, in front of the giant headstone, under the name of my mom's brother who died at just 18 years old from leukemia. It hits me in a way that I never before grasped that my Granny lost a child, a live one. And I wonder how she did it. How she buried him, how she moved on from burying him.

Earlier that week, my husband and I went to the funeral home to discuss what to do with our baby's remains, sign the documents, and pay the $500 required to turn her to ash. We were taken by one of the funeral directors into a room decorated lavishly in mahogany furniture and handed a huge binder. While the director was off printing the 10-page contract for us to sign, we flipped through the book looking at photos of small white coffins with tiny crosses or flowers etched into the wood. There were a surprising array of urns for children that looked like small ceramic piggy banks in various baby-centric forms: block letters, teddy bears, cute elephants, bows and cars and dolls. I had a visceral reaction to these images and knew that this was not for us. These vessels were for people who have held their babies, who have seen their babies play with teddy bears and elephants or cars and dolls. It would feel false to place her in something so indicative of a child's life when she had never had one. And besides, I wanted to be able to see an elephant or a piggy bank or a teddy bear down the road one day and not immediately think of an urn. I wanted to keep those images as things that are nice and happy — for me, but also for my son, who still has a childhood to live with me as his mother.

When the director came back in, I asked her, "Don't you have something more … simple?" After some hemming and hawing and a few mental calculations, she seemed to concede to the fact that I would not be placing my baby inside a ceramic elephant, and she informed me that the remains were actually provided in a small velvet bag and that if we wanted, we could just go with that, free of charge. I jumped at the small velvet bag.

Kneeling in front of the hole I've just dug, I think of my granny and how she probably had to go in and pick out a casket for her son and decide what wood grain best represented him. I open up the burgundy velvet pouch for the first time since it was filled with my baby's remains to find that contained within is another pouch, a plastic one, tied up with a metal ring. I am not prepared for this. I try to pull the ring off but it doesn't budge. I try to rip a hole in the top of the plastic bag, but this is no flimsy Ziploc bag; this is made of sturdier stuff, and I can't even put a dent in it.

My dad gets off the bench as he sees me struggling and comes beside me, pulling his car key out of his jacket pocket. Once again, I feel grateful he's shown up for me in all of this.

When I was lying in hospital, having just been told that our baby had no heartbeat, he showed up and he held me while I cried, and even cried with me. That was not something he had often been able to do in my life — bear witness to my pain — but I needed it so badly that day and I think he knew that. I think he needed it, too.

He takes the bag from me and starts forcefully sawing at the plastic with the edge of the key. Suddenly, the bag bursts open and a puff of grey ash spurts out and gets all over our hands. We both have an instinctive reaction to get the ashes off our hands and we start brushing frantically. It's not a nice feeling to have a dead person's ashes explode on your hands, even if they are a baby's. But then I can see it hit him at the same time it hits me without saying a word: this is the closest either of us will ever come to holding this much-desired baby girl. And so the frantic brushing stops and instead becomes a loving, gentle caress to transfer the ashes from our skin into the hole. I empty the rest of the bag into the earth, and then my mom helps me remove the daisy from its plastic container. She kneels down beside me, and together we place the flower on top of the tiny mound of grey, making sure to press it low enough so that there is enough earth to cover the roots of the plant. As if it will matter. We fuss around with the soil, smoothing it back and forth over the daisy, making sure the ground around it is neat and tidy, extending each second of this task before there is no more left to be done and it becomes more final than it already is.

We stand up, me between my parents, all of us staring down at the white daisy. I feel like I can hear a thought course back and forth between them: *We are burying our baby's baby.*

I realize then my husband is still standing behind us, apart, and even though his energy is telling me that he wants to be left alone, I pull him into our fold so that he can be held up, too, if just for a moment, between us all. I feel his body shudder ever so slightly, a mixture of grief and release and the cold air that's starting to bite at us. He doesn't speak the entire time we are there, from the time we arrive to the time we leave. But because I know him, this doesn't bother me. I know that this is how he needs to grieve and this is how he needs to cope — with us, but on his own. So I grant him the space to keep his thoughts and his words to himself, to hide the pangs in his heart under a blanket of silence.

This is the part where the priest or the minister or the rabbi says something biblical and profound before everyone can leave to go back to the assigned meeting place for quiet conversation and party sandwiches. But since this is not even a real funeral, I have decided that role is mine. It makes me think of a scene at the end of *Steel Magnolias* when Sally Field's character yells and cries to her friends, after just burying her daughter, that she is lucky because she got to be there when "that beautiful creature" came into the world and she got to be there when she left it. I think to myself, *Yeah, I get you, Sally Field*. I get the feeling of being all at once sad and grateful because I got the most special parts of this baby, just for me and me alone, because I am her mother. My parents, my husband, they have lost something, no doubt. But for them it's different. For them, they've lost the potential of a baby. What I've lost is more tangible: while I never held my baby girl in my arms, never kissed her forehead or touched my nose to hers, I held her in me, in my body and in my soul. I carried her in my heart, as E.E. Cummings wrote. She was as much a part of me as my blood and my organs that had housed her. I knew her. *I know her*. I know she would have been funny. I know she would have been a spitfire and a handful in her own right, just like her older brother. I know she would have been sassy, and girly, in all the best ways. I know she would have been my sidekick and my best friend even though some people say you're not supposed to be friends with your children. But we would have been. And how do you un-know that? How do you explain to your insides that this creature you were lucky enough to bring into this world and lucky enough to see out of this world is not actually, anymore, your baby? You can't.

This idea helped me to choose the words I speak over her makeshift daisy grave in lieu of a priest or a minister or a rabbi. Not so much as a memorial, but as a declaration to myself, my husband, my parents, to the Chinese ancestors and anyone else who is listening. *To her.*

I unfold the piece of paper I hastily scribbled on earlier, knowing I wouldn't remember the lines in the moment. They are words I heard many years ago as a small child, sitting in a circle on the carpet in a classroom during book time as a teacher read them aloud. They are by Robert Munsch, and I had no idea then that they were written from a place of invisible grief.

I clear my throat and read aloud, a little bit self-consciously because I'm not sure what everyone will think of my choice:

"I'll love you forever, I'll like you for always, as long as I'm living, my baby you'll be."

No one responds. Maybe it's because they don't need to. Instead, they let the greatest truth I've ever known and ever spoken hang in the air above us, filling the silent space between us and around us as we stand there for those last few moments. I let the yellow sunshine envelop me. I let it hit all the dark places inside of me. And then we tacitly agree that the funeral is done and walk down the slight hill back toward our cars. Once we reach the road, the veil seems to lift and it's as though we are allowed to make noise again because we've left that sacred space. We talk about what we all have to do with the rest of our days, me treading carefully as I move down the incline so as not to pull at my still-healing stitches. We all hug. My mom mentions what a beautiful day it is and we all turn our heads up to the sun, the blue sky. It really is a beautiful day. She gets in her car to drive back home; my dad heads off to work.

Before my husband and I climb into our car, I take one last look up the hill to the white daisy grave. I let myself believe that my baby is not gone even though we just buried her body. She is still here, around me, because of me.

And somehow, someway, I will find her again.

4

THE STARS IN MY SKY

Neil McKay

THERE ARE MANY THINGS I will never get to do with my son, Jacob. I'll never get to teach him how to throw and catch a ball. I'll never get to teach him how to ride a bike. I'll never get to take him to his first Leafs game.

I'll never get to do any of these things with him because Jacob passed away at birth.

In 2014, my wife, Haylie, and I decided we wanted to start a family. A short time later, we were pleased to find out she was pregnant. Fortunately for us, this process happened quite quickly.

We did all the normal things that expectant parents do. We shared our happy news with family and friends, the nursery was painted, the crib and change table were bought, and so on. We also attended many medical appointments. It was a very happy and exciting time for us. My wife felt lots of kicks and pokes, and I was lucky to be able to feel the odd one here or there as well. I fell into the habit of talking to our baby by speaking to Haylie's belly.

Our excitement grew as we neared the second ultrasound appointment. We planned to find out our baby's gender. Neither of us could wait until the delivery to find out the sex. We went to the ultrasound, eagerly antici-pating that we would soon know whether our family would grow through the addition of a little boy or girl. Our baby's heartbeat was strong and the baby was moving around a lot. Unfortunately, due to all the movement, or so we thought, the ultrasound technician was unable to get the required view in order to determine the baby's gender. Although this was disappointing, I was still excited to get a sneak peek at our baby.

Haylie was upset, though. She hadn't liked the technician's demeanour toward us. In addition, she had a feeling that something was wrong with our baby. The ultrasound technician had asked if she had been sick or dehydrated lately, as the amniotic fluid was lower than it should have been. I reassured her that everything was fine; we had just seen our baby moving around all over the place and the heartbeat was strong.

A day or two after the ultrasound, our family doctor called and put Haylie on bedrest. We were referred to a neonatal specialist.

Haylie stayed home, rested, and consumed a lot of water in hopes this would help with the low amniotic fluids the doctor had mentioned. In general, I'm not a person who worries about much, so I felt positive about our situation. The heartbeat, the movement, the pokes in the belly. *It had to be okay, and it would all work out,* I thought. I shared my positive feelings with my wife in an attempt to reassure her.

After an agonizing wait of several days, we went to the hospital. First up was another ultrasound, to be followed by a meeting with our neonatal specialist. Haylie went in for the ultrasound and I was invited into the room about 45 minutes later. Once again, I was pleased to see the baby moving around. The heart was beating strongly, which was comforting to me. Our baby was a fighter. A Lionheart. Once again, a gender determination could not be made.

After the ultrasound, we were called into a room to meet with the specialist. Of course, I knew that there was some issue, but I thought it would be something small that could be dealt with during the pregnancy. Little did I know my optimism was about to be entirely crushed.

The specialist introduced himself and got right to the point. "Your baby has something called bilateral renal agenesis, or Potter's syndrome. This is what is termed a lethal diagnosis."

It is impossible to put into words the feelings you have when your world has just been shattered. Going into that appointment, losing our baby wasn't something I had even considered, and now it was our unavoidable reality.

Essentially, Potter's syndrome meant our baby wasn't properly developing kidneys or a bladder. We were told this happens in about 1 in 5,000 pregnancies and there was nothing that could be done to help our baby. Nothing at all.

This was obviously hard for us to accept. As a father, your job is to love and protect your child, and I was useless in this situation. Completely powerless. Love doesn't conquer all.

We were given the opportunity to meet with a counsellor, who went over the available options. I had no trouble making up my mind once all of the options were presented to us. However, given that my wife would have to physically go through whatever we decided, I knew she should have the final say in the matter. Fortunately, we were both on the same page. Neither of us could bear the thought of terminating the pregnancy at this point. We still wanted the opportunity to hold our child.

We would have our baby.

Our families knew we had the appointment with the specialist that day and were anxiously awaiting an update. We ended up being at the hospital for a long time, and upon returning home we had the unenviable task of informing our families that the worst-case scenario would be coming true. These were tremendously difficult phone calls to make.

That evening, Haylie and I continued to try to come to terms with what had just transpired. It was, of course, impossible. Many tears were shed between us as we comforted one another. My wife made a poignant observation when she said, "Everybody is talking about the baby like they're already gone, and they're not."

As part of that conversation, she had the idea we should do things together as a family while our baby was still physically with us. With this in mind, we bought books and read to our baby every night. Some of these were really hard to get through, but we managed. I'm really glad Haylie thought of this as a way to help us process our grief, because I'll remember and cherish these moments for the rest of my life.

The next weekend, I ran my first marathon in Toronto, and the thought of our child was never out of my mind. Since then, running has reminded me of this time in my life and has provided a bond between me and my child.

After the race, we returned to our hometown of London, Ontario, and decided to stop at Springbank Park, a favourite spot of ours. Haylie wanted to get some pictures taken of her while she was pregnant. The vibrant fall leaves provided a beautiful background. We took some really nice photos, one of which is displayed in our home. The spot where we took that particular picture has special meaning for me whenever I pass by it. It always reminds me of the time that my wife and I were still physically together with Jacob.

We continued to deal with a full range of emotions surrounding our impending loss. About a week after the diagnosis, we found ourselves in the hospital again, this time awaiting the birth of our child, at 22 weeks' gestation.

The process started on Wednesday evening and continued into Thursday. Originally, we'd planned on going through this experience on our own, but in the end we felt our parents deserved the opportunity to meet their grandchild.

In some instances of Potter's syndrome, the baby will survive the birth. However, due to the amniotic fluids being low, their lungs do not develop enough to sustain life beyond a few precious moments.

We were still able to hear our baby's heartbeat throughout the birthing process as my wife and baby were monitored. We had planned on having the monitor on throughout, but Haylie decided we should turn it off when labour kicked into high gear. As our baby was expected to pass away during the birth, it would have made things even more difficult if we had known exactly the moment it transpired.

On the afternoon of October 23, 2014, our baby was born. As expected, stillborn. His gender was finally revealed and we officially welcomed Jacob Carter McKay into our family, into our arms, and completely into our hearts. It was an amazing experience to hold my son for the first time.

I was proud of my wife for being so strong throughout all of this. While this experience was the hardest thing I'd been through, my wife also had to handle the physical act of labour in addition to the draining emotional aspects. She is incredible.

I was also really proud of my son. I'm thankful I had the opportunity to hold him, to kiss him, and to tell him how much I loved him. While Jacob had a physical issue that prevented his survival, he was perfect in every other way. Jacob weighed exactly one pound, a tiny little guy who has had a huge impact on my life. My little Lionheart.

After his birth, we were given time to spend together as a family. We read a book that we had saved for his birth. We took many pictures. We had plaster casts made of his tiny feet. We listened to some songs together. But most of all, we held Jacob and loved him. We also gave him some gifts. We had brought along a few different items, not knowing if we would be having a boy or a girl. In the end, I gave him a little set of hockey gloves with the Canadian national team logo on them.

After spending seven hours together with Jacob, we were left with the impossible task of saying goodbye. Accompanied by a nurse, we brought Jacob to what is known as the "quiet room." We said goodbye to our boy and left him to be cared for by others. We had just gone through the birthing process but we did not get to bring our little boy home. We took the memory box with us, which contained mementos from the day: his foot casts, some clothes he wore, and the measuring tape that told us how long he was. We headed home. I felt the need to drive slowly in order to protect the items and memories that were housed in that little box.

I couldn't protect Jacob, but I could protect his memories.

I helped my wife into our house as she carried Jacob's box in. I returned to the car to gather our things. As I unloaded the car, I looked up to see a sky full of stars. The sky from that particular night has stuck with me always. I took those stars as a sign of a greater connection between my son and me.

Over the next days and weeks, we would try to come to terms with what had happened. We sought out the stories of others who had experienced similar situations to ours. We were shocked to find out just how common these occurrences are. As my wife remarked at the time, "It's amazing that any healthy babies are born, considering how much can go wrong."

I vividly recall waking up one morning with tears in my eyes. I had been crying in my sleep, something that until that moment would've seemed impossible to me.

My wife and I continued to lean on one another for comfort and support, and we had our families available to help us, too. This experience brought us closer together as a couple, which, I would subsequently come to learn, is not always the case.

As an elementary school teacher, I was apprehensive about returning to work. I wasn't sure how I would feel being around children so soon after losing my own child.

In preparation for my return after 10 days away, my class of grade five students had been told that something bad had happened and that I might be sad when I returned. My students were happy to have me back, which was nice. Somewhat surprisingly, they didn't ever ask me why I had been gone.

My co-workers were happy to have me back as well. They had all been made aware of what had happened. Many of them had offered condolences via email in response to an email I had sent out. Only a couple of co-workers addressed what had happened in person. It was nice to have support from those who took the time to speak with me, but I understand why a number of other people didn't. Before this happened, I would never have said anything to a person in my situation. It's hard to know what to say and, realistically, pretty uncomfortable, as you may be worried about causing further upset. I can't speak on behalf of all people who've lost a child, but for me, I've become comfortable with speaking about the loss. It gives me comfort and pride to be able to speak about Jacob. The other thing that was notable was how many people came forward to share their own losses of children.

As far as being around kids went, it wasn't at all problematic. In fact, there was one encounter with a small child that was quite meaningful. I was walking down a nearly empty hallway at school when a kindergarten student approached me and got my attention. He said, "This is yours," and handed me a small handmade pumpkin he had found on the ground. When I turned it over, I saw it said "Daddy" on the other side. Clearly not mine, but an interesting coincidence.

As time wore on, my wife and I continued to grieve. We had discussed getting a pet when we were in the hospital and soon welcomed a new cat into our home. Winnie was by no means a replacement for our son, but having that warmth, an outlet for love in our home, offered some aid in our healing.

Haylie and I would occasionally spend time with the items from Jacob's memory box, either together or on our own. In particular, I liked to smell the clothes he had worn, as they smelled like him. My wife also made a beautiful baby book to commemorate our son, a book I would look at many times in the months that followed his birth.

How is it that you get over the loss of a child?

You don't.

I will mourn my son for the rest of my life and hold him in my heart until it stops beating. I still say good morning and goodnight to Jacob every single day. Sometimes, I will just be driving to work and he will appear in my thoughts. It can make me feel a little sad, but I like that he's there. I like that he is still very much present in my life today.

When we were in the hospital with Jacob, many people talked to us about how we would be back in the hospital before we knew it welcoming another baby into our family. This was both helpful and hurtful. Haylie summed it up well when she said, "I don't want another baby. I want Jacob."

As time went on, though, we decided that we wanted to try again. Once we had the medical go-ahead, we tried, and soon we were fortunate once again to be expecting.

Obviously, based on the outcome of our first pregnancy, the second one was somewhat stressful. It was considered high-risk and my wife was placed under the care of a specialist. This was helpful, as it allowed us to get extra support. We had an additional ultrasound around the time that Potter's syndrome becomes apparent in order to rule it out and give us some peace of mind.

Before we knew it, we were back in the specialist's office to get the results of that ultrasound. We had been told the chances of Potter's syndrome happening again were essentially nonexistent, but still, until you hear all is okay, there is always that tiny seed of doubt. We ended up getting the results in the same room where we had received Jacob's diagnosis. This did not go unnoticed.

Thankfully, our doctor told us good news: the kidneys were developing. He mentioned a couple of markers that were present on the heart and brain, but quickly assured us that these were nothing to worry about. He also revealed to us the gender of our second child. A little girl.

Around midnight on October 16, 2015, my wife woke me up to let me know her water had broke. As we left our home, I noticed the sky was clear and many stars were visible in the sky. I knew that Jacob was with us that night.

Exactly 51 weeks to the day of Jacob's birth, we welcomed a beautiful little girl into our lives, Hadley Isobel Jane McKay. We could not have been happier. I made sure to stop at the door of the quiet room at one point after Hadley's birth. I paused, placed my hand on the door, and remembered my son.

Things were going well with Hadley in the days that followed her birth, although she had some jaundice our doctor was monitoring. In addition to welcoming Hadley into our family, we had been making plans to celebrate what would have been Jacob's first birthday.

We brought Hadley to our doctor to follow up on her jaundice and she advised us to immediately bring Hadley to emergency, where they would assess her. Our doctor was concerned her jaundice was getting worse. She felt that Hadley might need to be put under phototherapy lights in order to reduce the jaundice. The emergency doctors took Hadley's blood and told us that they were checking her bilirubin levels, which indicated the severity of jaundice.

Suddenly, hospital staff rushed into our room and whisked Hadley down the hall. She was immediately placed under phototherapy lights and we were told her levels were exceptionally high. She was in grave danger. This occurred 364 days after the loss of our son.

Hadley was admitted to the Paediatric Critical Care Unit where she underwent a double-volume blood transfusion. We stood beside her bed as her heroic doctors and nursing staff manually circulated her blood. The concern was that Hadley could develop something called kernicterus, which leads to cerebral palsy.

Our plans to celebrate Jacob's birthday were put on hold. On his first birthday, we were in hospital with our brave little girl. We would stay in the hospital with Hadley for a week or so. We had already had a rare-occurrence health issue with Jacob and here we were again. A bilirubin level as high as Hadley's was also extremely rare. *How could we be struck twice like this?*

At one point during Hadley's hospitalization, we visited the hospital chapel. I'm not at all religious, but it was nice and quiet and a peaceful spot to escape to for a while. I did not pray to God. Instead, I asked Jacob to take care of his little sister, and he did.

Hadley made a full recovery. She is now a perfectly healthy, very happy, busy two-year-old. She is smart, strong, and beautiful and is an exceptionally cool little girl. She is so much fun and I love her so much.

The following week, we celebrated Jacob's birthday back in Springbank Park at the site where we had taken the pictures after the marathon. We released some balloons at that spot, returned home, had cupcakes, and spent time remembering our little boy. It is a tradition we have followed every year since his birth. He would be three now.

Jacob has an uncanny ability to appear when I need him. Out of millions of songs in the world, there are four I associate with Jacob. There have been countless times when I have heard one of those songs when I needed a little extra strength. Jacob is just there in those times. I can't explain it, but I happily accept it.

It can be hard when I think about the fact that I lost a son. However, these moments don't always hurt. I'm just glad, whether or not they are painful, that I still have them, because they keep him close to me. Mostly, when I think of Jacob I'm happy. He lives on in many different ways: in the stars in the sky, in the lyrics of the four songs, and in the kilometres I run, and despite the lack of a physical presence, he's the greatest big brother and the most amazing son.

When it comes time for the World Junior Hockey Championship or the Olympics, I place his hockey gloves on the shelf where his ashes rest and I know my son is watching those games with me. Father and son, together, inseparable forever. My boy.

I began my story by writing about all of the things I will never get to do with my son. However, I prefer to look at what I gained through my experience. A bond that will never be broken between my son and me. Special memories I will always hold of places we were together as a family, of books, and of songs that remind me of him.

There is a 24-hour ultramarathon run in my hometown every year. By coincidence, the race passes by our spot in Springbank Park where we go every year to celebrate our little boy's birthday. This year, I ran this race in honour of Jacob and Hadley in order to raise money for childrens' health initiatives. I passed by Jacob's spot around 60 times during that 24-hour period. I acknowledged him quietly on each lap. As night fell, the sky was clear and the stars abundant. During my lowest point, about 13 hours into the race and the only time I questioned whether I would be able to complete it, three of my "Jacob songs" played consecutively.

Rather remarkable, since my playlist was on random and there are hundreds of songs on it. I finished the race.

When I first considered sharing our story, Haylie and I discussed the pros and cons. On the one hand, keeping Jacob's story to ourselves, our family, and our friends would keep it personal. Insulated: our boy and us. In the end, though, we decided others could benefit from our loss, from our pain. We knew that when we navigated our way through the loss of a child, we took comfort in the stories of others. We hope that by sharing our story, we can help others through the loss of a child. Because you need help to get through it, to persevere, to come out the other side, and to go on. Losing a child is the hardest thing you will ever go through. Ever. You are not alone; we are many and we are strong.

As I put the finishing touches on this essay late one Saturday night, my wife walked into the room. She had something to tell me. She happened to notice that the sky was full of stars.

In 2014, I lost a child but gained so much. In the past year, I've had a number of opportunities to share my son's story. When you lose a child, you are no less proud of them, but you do miss out on the opportunity to talk about them, as it makes many people feel uncomfortable. I'm thankful for the opportunity to speak about Jacob.

More recently, our family became complete with the birth of our younger daughter, Eleni. She has brought even more warmth into our lives. Adding snuggles and smiles in the way that only a newborn can. Haylie and I have been fortunate enough to have three amazing, beautiful children.

My story is not a sad one. I have a complete family. I will forever wish that I could hold all three of my children at the same time. Play in the backyard with them all, share the smiles and excitement of Christmas morning. Watch them grow into the people we all hope our children become. For me, that won't ever be physically possible. However, our children exist where we hold them. For some, that is in our arms; for all, it is in our hearts. I love you, Haylie. I love you, Jacob. I love you, Hadley. I love you, Eleni.

5

IT'S JUST BAD LUCK

Amelie Roberge

I HAVE BEEN PREGNANT five times, but have only one child. I always wanted kids. My sister and I were avid babysitters (not Babysitter Club level, but we could dream), and I always enjoyed the company of young kids. I believed the hype that popular culture and TV specials teach kids — that getting pregnant is dangerously easy. As I got older, my friends and family began having babies on purpose. It seemed just that simple for all of them.

My husband and I decided not to "try" for a baby; rather, we would not do anything to actively prevent it. I tried to be relaxed and cool about the whole thing, but I was so excited at the thought of us as parents. I knew my husband would make the best dad. I couldn't wait to snuggle a baby I didn't have to return to its rightful caregiver afterward. I like to think of myself as a realist, but when I pictured myself pregnant and then with the baby, all I saw was bliss — fuzzy-screen, living-in-the-clouds bliss. I had one specific fantasy that makes no sense when I reflect back on it. I would be on maternity leave on a beautiful summer's day, sitting outside in my backyard, lying on a lounge chair (that I don't own), drinking an iced tea (which I don't like) and reading a novel while my baby slept (ha) in a Pack 'n Play covered in a mosquito net. No idea where this came from, but it was a vision I kept returning to.

The first time I had a miscarriage, I had no idea I was pregnant. I had only recently gone off the pill and my period was very irregular. I had been on birth control for over a decade, so I fully expected my body to have a re-action to the change. I thought it was just a late, heavy period, but the bleeding didn't stop. When I went to see my doctor, he told me that I had had a miscarriage, and for the first time I felt my heart fall. He called it a chemical pregnancy, and I think he used that term to try to make me feel less attached to the life that was lost. It didn't help. I had never felt such a loss for someone I hadn't even met. But I buried myself in articles about how normal miscarriages are. They were reassuring. I grieved for what might have been and decided the timing hadn't been great, anyway. I mean, we had only recently gotten married and our apartment was so tiny. Now we had more time to prepare, right? One little chemical pregnancy was no reason to get discouraged.

The second time I had a miscarriage, I knew I was pregnant. I was already deeply in love with the little life growing inside me. I am Jewish and there is a strong cultural superstition against celebrating babies before they are born. Basically, it comes down to not inviting the evil eye into your life. Many Jewish families choose not to have baby showers, decorate the nursery, or even select a name until the baby is actually born. Traditionally, you don't even say *mazel tov*, or congratulations, to a Jewish mother-to-be. My grandmother always said "*B'sha'ah tovah*," which means "In good time." The tradition runs pretty deep and I was raised that way; I learned super-stitions almost through osmosis. I notice it in my mom and sister, too. Not just about babies, either. Really, it's the idea that celebrating anything before it happens might cause something bad to happen instead.

Against all my superstitious cultural training, I started making plans right away. At least in my head — never out loud to anyone except my husband. Since the baby was due in January, I couldn't finish a particu-lar project at work. And since the baby was due in January, we probably couldn't travel at Christmas that year. Ridiculous mundane things like that.

I wasn't really worried about the pregnancy because — as all my read-ing had taught me — one miscarriage didn't mean anything: It's so normal! It's so common!

One day, at 11 weeks pregnant, I stopped at my favourite sandwich spot on my way home from work. I happily brought home a brisket sand-wich to eat completely guilt-free, thanks to the fact that I was eating for two. I was enjoying it so vividly, right before I went to the bathroom. And that's when I saw the blood. For the second time, I felt my heart fall. I tried to reassure myself that it was just spotting. I went to the hospital, just in case, and they confirmed that my hormone levels were lower than they should be. They said that if my levels continued to drop, it was a good indication that I would miscarry.

Miscarriages don't often get discussed. There are a lot of misconceptions about them. At least, there were in my mind. One of the things about miscarriages that people don't tell you is how long they last. I had always thought it was like in the movies. The woman feels a terrible pain in her stomach or falls down some stairs (I watched a lot of soap operas growing up), loses the baby, and then rests a bit. In reality, miscarriages can last more than a week, and women often carry on with their lives while having them. I felt silly that I didn't know this. I also, oddly, felt a surge a pride for womanhood in general — unbeknownst to me, I have probably encountered countless women who just had to go ahead and deal with life and work and family while losing a life inside them. We are so strong.

Another thing people don't tell you is how helpless you feel when the doctor says you will likely miscarry. There is nothing you can do to try to save your baby. Nothing. It's one of the worst feelings in the whole wide world. From the moment you find out you are pregnant, every instinct inside you says to protect your baby. But all you can do is just wait and see if the bleeding gets worse and if your hormone levels drop.

And while I felt strength in womanhood through it all, I also felt disappointment in modern Western medicine. I couldn't understand how we could put pigs' hearts in human beings to save lives, but hadn't figured out how to stop a miscarriage from happening.

The taxi ride home from the hospital felt like it took forever. Like time had stopped. It's an odd memory for me now. I know I was there. I remember staring out the window while this hollow feeling crept into the pit of my stomach. I remember not saying a word to my husband for the entire ride. I knew if I looked at him he would just have all this sadness and concern in his eyes, and I couldn't take it. I remember feeling completely numb. That was the moment when I started questioning if there was something wrong with me. Maybe I wasn't going to be able to have a child. Maybe this sadness would never go away.

When I started talking about my experiences to other women, they shared their own experiences of miscarriages with me. I had known about a few in my family, but suddenly great aunts, second cousins, and old friends of the family were messaging me to tell me about their losses. It was kind of amazing. If miscarriages are so common, then why do we hide them from each other? Why do we feel like miscarriages are something we should be ashamed of? It helped me feel normal and hopeful again to talk to other women about their experiences, and I can never thank them enough for that.

The third time I became pregnant I was excited and petrified at the same time. I didn't want to let myself get too invested, because I knew how quickly my happiness could turn into devastation. Against my logical brain, I went back to my deeply ingrained superstitions. I didn't really think that planning for my previous pregnancy had caused the miscarriage, but I was starting to believe that, at the very least, it couldn't hurt to try a little harder to ward off the evil eye. When I told my grandmother I was pregnant again, she said, "Oh, that's wonderful. I love you. Now we never speak of it again until it comes."

But, as usual when it came to my pregnancies, it was impossible to squash my excitement. I couldn't help but fall madly and instantly in love with the person growing inside me. I decided I could try to ward off the evil eye in other ways. Every time I went to the bathroom, I prayed that I wouldn't see blood. Seriously. Every single time. I wouldn't have a baby shower, and I definitely wouldn't announce it on social media. I didn't even tell my closest friends at first. Instead, I made coffee at the office every morning and then inconspicuously poured it down the drain. I was incredibly cautious with everything I did throughout the pregnancy — so cautious, in fact, that I encountered many unhelpful comments from people, like "Relax, women have been having babies forever" and "Women used to plough the fields right up until giving birth."

People have no idea what you have gone through before, and many assume that having babies is so natural that all these precautions women take nowadays are superfluous. They are not. I admit I was anxious. I was *this* close to buying my own fetal heart monitor a bunch of times, and for half a second was concerned that cheering too loudly at a Medieval Times Dinner and Tournament could hurt the baby.

But I was also beyond happy with every passing week. The baby grew and I grew and, at 30 weeks, I stopped praying every time I went to the bathroom. I even agreed to let my friends throw me a baby shower, albeit very close to my due date. I believed everything was going to be okay because I had made it this far without incident. Those other two times were obviously just bad luck, I told myself, and I was totally normal and could finally relax. So, of course, that's when I saw the blood. My heart fell.

I didn't know what to do. It was Passover and I was visiting my parents in Ottawa, along with my sister and her two children. My husband had taken the train up with me but had headed home earlier because I had some extra time off and I wanted to spend it with my family. I was a four-hour drive away from him and my doctor in Toronto. My mom tried to keep me calm while rushing me to the hospital. She is one of the strongest people I know, and she had this look in her eyes that I had seen only once before, when my father had had a stroke. I was freaking out.

When we arrived, they immediately put a fetal monitor on me. I don't think I actually breathed from the moment I saw the blood at my parents' house to the moment I heard my baby's heartbeat at the hospital. They didn't know what was wrong (a recurring theme with doctors, I've discovered), but they said that everything was going to be okay. My son was going to be okay. I held on to that. I could breathe. The hospital in Ottawa wanted me to stay, but I wanted to be with my husband and treated by my OB/GYN, so they gave my mother a list of every hospital between Ottawa and Toronto and said I could go home as long as she drove me. We had a road trip I'm sure neither of us will ever forget, but happily, we didn't end up needing the list of hospitals.

When I saw my doctor back in Toronto, I was put on bedrest. Admittedly, I was kind of excited that I would wait out the rest of my pregnancy with my Netflix account and some ice cream. Also, I had heard a lot about *Dance Moms* and thought this was finally my moment to watch it.

My son had other plans. He was born just a week later and six weeks premature — early, but healthy. I always tell him now that he kind of saved me, because when I rushed to the hospital (again) it was because I was bleeding (again). The hospital admitted me to the antepartum wing, which I had never known existed. I discovered a whole ward full of very pregnant women trying not to go into labour. My doctor said I would need to stay there for the rest of my pregnancy. This was not the Netflix and bedrest that I had been picturing. It felt kind of depressing.

I was there for only one night before I went into labour. I always say Ben was like, "Nope, this sucks. Mama, I got this. I'll be fine. I'm coming out now."

Ben had to stay in the neonatal intensive care unit for two weeks to grow a little more and learn how to eat before we could bring him home. While it was heartbreaking to be away from him, my son was going to be okay. That's really all I cared about. The day we brought him home, which was supposed to be the day of his now-cancelled baby shower, I put him in his bassinet, which was next to my bed, and we both fell asleep right away, holding hands. It was the best sleep I had had in weeks.

Now that Ben was home and I was on maternity leave, none of the earlier problems seemed to bother me. I never lived out the lounge-chair-and-iced-tea fantasy, but it was one of the happiest years of my life.

I became pregnant again when Ben was two years old. And, like some kind of perverse optimist, I wasn't very worried about having a miscarriage again. I had had a successful pregnancy. I had a son. My body would know exactly what to do this time, right? Sure, I still prayed every time I went to the bathroom, but I swear it had worked the first time around. I had early ultrasounds to make sure everything was going okay. Everything was under control. And then one night, when I was 12 weeks pregnant, I went to the bathroom and there was the blood. My heart fell again and again. The familiar feeling of sinking and not being able to breathe returned.

I had to go to the hospital alone this time because now we had a child at home and my husband had to stay with him. The ultrasound was inconclusive. My hormone levels weren't great but they also weren't terrible, and it could just be spotting this time. I couldn't believe the wave of hope I was feeling — I almost felt guilty that I had assumed the worst. Almost. I remained skeptical. Part of me knew what was really happening. I could feel it.

The bleeding got worse and I went to see my obstetrician, who confirmed I was having a miscarriage. This time, I would have to have a dilation and curettage (D&C) procedure. It was awful. Finding the words to describe how I felt at that moment feels impossible. I was despondent, and the loss of hope for this other baby was physically painful. I was angry. I blamed a lot of factors; the most hurtful of all was myself. I didn't want to admit it, but the timing of the second child had been a bit stressful. I found out I was pregnant on exactly the same day I received a promotion at work. The thought of paying for two kids in daycare seemed to be taking the joy out of this pregnancy for me and my husband. I was mad at us for not being only overjoyed by the pregnancy, and I felt guilty about it at the same time.

A D&C is sometimes an outpatient procedure. You wait in a surgical waiting room until they call your number. You lie down on the table completely naked under your robe, and then you wake up wearing unfamiliar underwear. It's completely unsettling. Maybe it was also because I had, fortunately, never had surgery before, and when I had Ben, labour had come on so quickly that I couldn't use any kind of pain management. So I had never been out of it quite like this before, and I didn't like how it felt. I also didn't know how to feel about the D&C itself. On one hand, I liked the finality of it — my miscarriages seemed to last forever and this procedure expedited everything. But it also felt like my miscarriages were a much bigger deal healthwise than I had been allowing myself to believe. After it was done, I ate the arrowroot cookie and drank the juice they gave me and went home. In another silent taxi ride with my husband.

My third miscarriage. I didn't want anyone's sympathy. I didn't want anyone telling me that if I really wanted another child I could have one. I didn't want anyone telling me about all my options. I just wanted to be left alone. But I had a son, so that wasn't possible. And as cliché as this sounds, he was the best medicine. Taking care of another human and trying my best to keep him from noticing that his mama was sick really made me move on more quickly. At least I thought it did. I decided this sort of thing happens to everyone and I had so much good in my life. I decided to focus on my perfect son, my loving husband, and all the other people and things I loved in my life. I tried to force myself to get over it. I had to. There was no other option.

The following year I became pregnant again, and again I pretended to do the whole "Let's not get excited" routine. I told my close friends and family, since these were the people I would get support from whether I was sharing my happiness or my sadness. And, just like I had before, I uncontrollably loved this little thing growing inside me. I didn't bother praying before going to the bathroom since it hadn't worked the last time, plus God and I were on the outs a bit. I had always believed in God in a complicated I-also-believe-in-science way. I believed that bad things happening to good people didn't negate what I felt was my own personal relationship with my faith. But after the third miscarriage, I wasn't sure about anything anymore.

I also didn't make any plans. I know — I always say I won't and then it ends up happening. During my last pregnancy, I had looked into part-time daycare that my son could attend while I was home with the new baby. This was very practical, as Toronto daycares are notoriously difficult to get into. I got on a waiting list, and months after the third miscarriage, they contacted me about the spot.

And then one day, when I was 13 weeks pregnant, I saw the blood. My heart fell, and this time, it fell the furthest. It was like my heart had never truly recovered from the other miscarriages and now it was too far down an abyss to ever make its way back up. My miscarriages seemed to be getting progressively worse: later in the pregnancy, more blood loss each time, greater recovery time each time. This was the worst one: the most blood, the deepest sadness, and the greatest anger. It was all just too much. I needed a wheelchair to get from the taxi to the hospital room. This one sent me to therapy. I knew I needed to talk with someone who didn't love me, someone who could just listen and not worry about me.

And it helped. My only experience with therapy up until this point had been one session I went to in university, and that had actually been a mix-up. I thought I was going to see an academic adviser, but she was a therapist and I had had a crazy year of family illness, moving across the world from my family, and the death of a loved one. The hour just flew by. That day, I realized even one session of talking about your feelings with a professional could do wonders for your outlook.

After all the miscarriages, I felt my whole being was different. I felt very, very angry and I didn't like it. I also didn't feel like I could fix it and go back to my old self on my own. But one of the best things therapy taught me was not to worry about going back to my old self. These miscarriages and having Ben early were traumatic events, and it was okay to call them that. Compounded trauma is real. It made sense that I would be a different person afterward — and that was okay. It didn't make my anger disappear, but it gave me the tools to understand that it was okay to be angry. That was very powerful.

My family doctor referred me to an infertility/multiple miscarriage specialist. I wasn't even sure I wanted to try to have another child anymore, but I didn't want to leave some kind of miracle solution out on the table. Maybe there was something wrong with my husband? Maybe I just needed the slightest bit more progesterone? Maybe this could all be fixed with one tiny pill? We went to the specialist. I had more than 15 vials of blood taken from me in one sitting, and my husband just a bit less. They did genetic tests for everything under the sun. For half a moment, they thought my husband might have an abnormal chromosome situation, and we couldn't believe there was a reason for all this loss we suffered. But upon second testing they discovered that he was normal. I was so disappointed in his normality. I went into the clinic nearly every morning to give more blood, along with what felt like nearly every over-30-year-old woman in Toronto. I had internal ultrasounds and cystoscopies. All to no avail.

In the end, they said there was nothing wrong with me. Nothing wrong with me. We just had terrible luck. This was not remotely comforting. I wanted an explanation — an explanation that came with a plan or a cure. This was just nothing. My anger with modern Western medicine grew and my anger with the world grew right along with it.

My husband and I discussed trying for another child, a lot. While I was going to the lab for daily tests, I was missing our daily family coffee shop visit and daycare drop-off. We usually all went together and it was a lovely part of our day. He wanted to know why I wanted another child after all I had gone through. Was it just how I had always imagined my family looking? He told me he could be content with just Ben and wanted to know if I could be, too. And then he said something that had never occurred to me before. He said that when I was in the hospital the last time, it was really scary for him, as my partner. That having me around and healthy as Ben's mom was more important than anything, and that I didn't seem to realize the effect that my hospital trips had had on him and Ben. Especially the last one.

That was enough for me. I asked the specialist if there was any way they could guarantee that if I became pregnant one more time — this time through in vitro fertilization — I would carry the baby to term. He said that there's never a guarantee. I decided that I couldn't risk losing another baby, for my sake and my family's sake.

That's when the shift in me really happened. I stopped worrying about having another child and about the spacing between siblings and about the cost of two children in daycare. A huge weight had been lifted from me and I felt almost like myself again. I realized that my life could be just fine with one child. No, not just fine. Great. And filled with the same amount of love and joy.

I have had four miscarriages in my life and they are all a part of me now. I will forever carry the love for those tiny beings I never got to meet. In a way, my story has become this sort of miraculous gift to me: the losses I've suffered have made me so aware of how lucky I am to be a mother. I think I might even be a more present parent because of it. I truly know how lucky I am to have my son, and that is a wonderful gift that all my other pregnancies have given me.

While my anger and grief haven't completely gone away, I feel like they have morphed me into a fierce woman of strength. I'm not sure I would have tapped into that had everything worked out exactly how I had imagined when I was 15. Now that I've had time to adjust, I'm not sure what I would change about my life. Though I could have lived without the sorrow, being Ben's mom is the best thing in my life. Honestly, he gets to have all of me and my husband, and I don't think I would want it any other way.

6

SPRING BIRTHDAY PARTIES

Melanie Orfus

LIKE MANY ANXIOUS CHILDREN, I had recurring nightmares when I was growing up. Some were silly, like the giant man made out of Kleenex tissues who chased me around my living room. Others felt so real I had to run to my parents' bed for comfort. One day, I asked my mom if what terrified me in my sleep might really happen. She gave me a hug and reassured me that nightmares could not come true. That night, I had one of my typical dreams that usually filled me with dread. But I wasn't afraid anymore. The story had changed.

I grew up in suburban Toronto with married parents and an older brother. As a little girl, I loved my teddy bears and dolls, often pretending to be their mother or teacher. I had a few close friends, whereas my brother always drew a crowd. As a moody teen, I often fought with my family; I spent more time outside the house or alone in my room than with them. I looked forward to leaving home and finding a new place for myself in university.

During my second year at Queen's, I met my husband, Isaac. We had an immediate connection, began dating, and remained devoted to each other throughout degrees, distance, and disaster. As it did for many, the tragedy of September 11, 2001, brought us closer together. We felt so fortunate to have found each other and promised never to end a conversation without saying "I love you." We got married in 2005.

In 2009, we moved to San Francisco. When Isaac's new job brought us the security of health insurance, we agreed to begin making our family. I found an obstetrician in the Bay Area and booked an appointment. A few weeks later, I received a clean bill of health and the go-ahead to try to conceive. For months, I took my temperature, tracked my cycles, and planned our intimacy accordingly. Nothing happened. Month after month, I was disheartened by my period, sometimes cruelly late. It was the enemy, and its monthly arrival the loss of a battle.

The stress of living in one of the most expensive cities in America weighed heavily on us both. Isaac's job was extremely demanding and he worked long hours. It had been difficult for me to secure a work visa because my job in health care was different in the United States than it had been in Canada. I could only work part-time and for a fraction of what I made back home. I felt unfulfilled in my career and I missed my friends in Toronto. I loved our adventures abroad, but the possibility of raising children in America intimidated me. Unlike my experience growing up in Canada, crime, politics, and racism could be prominent influences in our child's life. Even more disconcerting, at any time Isaac could be transferred to one of his firm's other locations around the world.

Due to stress, Isaac started having panic attacks and began talking in his sleep. Months of negative pregnancy tests had me doubting my own body. Isaac displayed only mild interest in planning for the baby, and I feared that even if I did get pregnant, I'd be handling most of the responsibilities alone.

One evening, Isaac mentioned buying a sailboat. He wanted to spend weekends sailing the Bay. I couldn't believe what he was suggesting — how could he think we could afford this? Where were his priorities? We had a terrible fight, and I left the apartment to cool off in the park across the street. When I returned, Isaac was packing a suitcase. I was stunned. Where was he going to go? And why did he want to leave? We talked for hours and came to a mutual understanding. We loved each other and were committed to our marriage. For the well-being of both of us, we needed to make changes. When an opportunity arose, I took a contract job in Toronto to earn us some more money. Isaac would be sent to his firm's office in London, England, for the summer. Our plans of having a baby would be put on hold.

It was early August and I'd just returned to Toronto after two romantic weeks with Isaac in Europe. We talked about still wanting a baby, and the timing of the recent trip made it possible to give it a shot. Weeks later, my period was late. I bought a test and spent that humid night tossing and turning anxiously, determined to wait until morning for the most accurate result. I didn't tell anyone that I hoped I was pregnant, including Isaac. I dismissed the nagging fear of disappointment and let myself fantasize to distract myself. I stared at my stomach in the mirror and thought about baby names.

At sunrise, I got up to take the test. Of the many I'd taken before, none had ever been positive. In my bathroom, I ripped open the box and threw away the instructions, not necessary for a veteran. After I finished peeing on the stick, I carefully set it on the edge of the sink and set a timer for two minutes. I returned to bed and listened to the sounds of Yonge Street below. Taxis honked and a faint siren screamed in the distance. When the timer went off, I jumped. I got up from bed, ran back to the sink, and froze. The little white stick said "Pregnant," transforming me into a mother.

It took a few seconds for this to sink in. When it did, pure exhilaration ran through my body. I enjoyed the greatest moment of my life in that tiny bathroom. I took a picture of the positive test to send to Isaac. I told the baby how excited her father would be to hear she was coming. We had many plans to make, including settling on a place to live.

Our cat, Ella, had dental surgery scheduled that same morning. I planned to call Isaac after I dropped her off at the vet when I got to work. It would be about lunchtime in London, and it would be better to call his work landline over his unreliable cell. Lately, it had been difficult to reach him. When his voice clicked onto the line he sounded professional, but then relaxed when he heard me. My heart was racing. I told him I had some news.

"I'm pregnant!" I exclaimed.

Silence.

I waited for him to absorb the news, twisting the phone cord between my fingers. When he said nothing, I asked him if he'd heard me. I repeated his name. Finally, he quietly said, "You shouldn't have told me at work." Click.

My heart and stomach dropped. I hung up the phone. I played with my wedding ring with my other hand. Then I cried the first of many painful tears to come. My soulmate and loving husband had behaved as if we were no more than strangers, on one of the happiest days of my life. As a woman, this changed me.

I didn't tell anyone except Naomi, my close friend and officemate, who had seen me devastated after the phone call. Isaac didn't contact me all day. After work, I picked up Ella at the vet and brought her home. Then I bought a few pregnancy books. Later in the evening, I tried calling him again but he didn't answer. I didn't know whether to worry or be enraged. After a restless sleep, I woke up to an email:

> Sorry I didn't speak to you last night, we drank pretty heavily. Anyway, I know you must have been freaked and/or hurt by my response to your phone call yesterday. I was just stressed at work and freaked out a bit. BUT, that is AWESOME FANTASTIC news. I have my fingers crossed that this comes true this time. Just took me some time to digest this news, but I really am happy!!! I sort of can't believe it! But, wow! Incredible!! I will call you at work later today as I want to see how Ella is doing.

I noticed that he didn't tell me he loved me, as he had the day before and every day prior for the past 11 years. I replied immediately and scolded him for how he had hurt me. His disappearance had been excruciating. He'd ruined a moment I had dreamed about my entire life. I reminded him that he needed to put the baby and me first. A few hours later, another email arrived in which he coolly stated he would call at 6:00 p.m. my time. My body went cold. My stomach was in knots. I left work crying again.

Right on time, my phone rang, and Isaac was on the other end. We were both quiet at first. I asked him how he could ignore me when I was finally carrying his child. What followed did not come from my husband and best friend. It was someone else; he sounded rehearsed and robotic.

"I don't love you anymore."

It was as simple as that.

Intense pain, shock, and desperation hit me. But I also felt disbelief and confusion. I knew things had been difficult, as I had imagined they would be at times in a marriage. But I was also certain he loved me. Beads of sweat poured down my back as I tried to understand what was happening. Unlike me, he was calm and clear as he kept repeating his cold, contrived refrain: "I don't love you anymore." I yelled and paced my un-air-conditioned apartment. I searched for the right phrase that would change his mind. I threatened him, saying that our baby wouldn't have his last name. But he didn't react, and his apathy infuriated me further. When he ended the call, I still had no answers. He was an ocean away in another land and I was alone with my baby. I had to figure out what to do.

I called close friends, who dropped everything to be with me. They helped me call my mom. I wasn't ready to face my dad, so I asked my mom to come see me, alone. This was not how I imagined delivering this wonderful news to her as a daughter. With my two best friends watching, I stood up and told her in one sentence that I was pregnant and Isaac had left me. I didn't know how she would react. She said she couldn't wait to meet her first grandchild. We hugged and cried.

My mom spent that night in my apartment, watching me try to sleep. She comforted me when I awoke crying. This was her first job as a grandmother. The next morning, we took a taxi up to my parents' house to tell my father. My parents were busy and stressed that summer, in the process of moving out of their home of 35 years. My dad was much older than my mom, with old-fashioned values and a quick temper. It was a rule growing up to avoid upsetting him. I had no idea what to expect from the stern man I had worked so hard to please as a daughter. He reacted with kindness, but also with practicalities. He told me to get a lawyer as he hugged me.

At five weeks pregnant, I cried frequently. When I was able to sleep, which was rare, I woke up with tears moistening my cheeks and pillows. An already picky eater, I had strong food aversions and no appetite. My mother did her best to feed me and keep me going. She also made it a priority to find me a more suitable place to live. We decided that the baby and I should move into the same building they were in so that I would have help.

When morning sickness began, it lasted all day and night. I became an expert at throwing up, doing it in alleyways, down sewers, and out of car doors. After throwing up on my shoes one morning, I tried harder to perfect my aim. I worried the baby wasn't getting enough nutrients. Fortunately, I had a supportive family doctor who did her best to reassure me everything was okay. She sent me for early ultrasounds before I saw an obstetrician. She referred me to a therapist specializing in early pregnancy. I noticed the office had the same chairs that Isaac and I had had in our home in California. I could not return.

People encouraged me to focus on the baby and my future. I was given a due date: April 22. I imagined spring birthday parties with fresh rain showers and flowers beginning to grow. I bought a few toys and took out the things I'd collected for my future baby over the years. Just recently, in London, I had bought a soft baby-blue rabbit. I tried to enjoy the idea of being able to choose everything myself, including the baby's first and last names.

Still, I missed Isaac terribly and the ache of his rejection was constant. He was adamant he didn't love me. I just as resolutely disbelieved him. I did desperate things, like sending him a picture of him kissing me weeks earlier on vacation. I forwarded him spontaneous texts he had sent me telling me he missed me and loved me. Everything had been fine. This did not make sense.

Meanwhile, Ella was still not recovering from dental surgery. After several examinations, it was discovered she had inoperable masses in her stomach. The veterinarian recommended I put her down. I was devastated and stumbled upon another layer of grief. So much was out of my control, everything changing and disappearing all at once.

Isaac loved Ella dearly. He agreed to talk over Skype so he could see her and say goodbye. Looking at each other face to face, even digitally, was painful. We cried over the loss that we knew was coming, and I could see the hard demeanour he'd carefully manufactured crumble beneath the weight. Sensing the opportunity to get answers, I pushed him with more questions. He struggled to regain his emotionless, calm facade. I threw questions at him. He shook his head again and again.

"Is there another woman? Are you addicted to gambling? Drugs? Did you commit a crime? Then what is it? Are you gay?"

He froze and I saw. I had thrown that last question in without thinking. It was never among the many theories I had considered. I thought about it for the first time in that moment.

"Are you gay?" I asked again quietly as he stared down.

"I think I might be."

I was shocked, but I also felt a tremendous amount of relief. Isaac quickly assured me he'd never acted upon these feelings. As I listened to him, my anger dissolved. He told me how scared he was and how he didn't know what to do. He still loved me, he promised over and over. He had panicked when he imagined hiding his secret from someone else he loved, our baby.

I felt his anguish as my own. I told him there was no need to hide. I still loved him, too. We would find a way to be a family. He was afraid, but I assured him I would be by his side. We were a team again, though we acknowledged it would be different. For several days, I enjoyed the fantasy of our accepting, alternative partnership. We spoke lovingly to each other again. Having spent the past few weeks in agony, it was like being in withdrawal from a drug and then having a relapse. I welcomed any new reality without considering the possible implications.

Despite my resistance to leaving this fantasy world, memories kept popping into my head, poking holes through Isaac's story. Even knowing what plagued him, I didn't understand how a planned pregnancy could trigger this kind of reaction. Even after my promised support, he was still evasive. He'd left the London office and was back in San Francisco, still refusing to come to Toronto. I thought about all the times I had not been able to reach him.

I remembered getting separated during a night out with friends in Los Angeles. We were catching a plane the next day and he wasn't answering his phone. He didn't arrive back at the hotel until 7:00 a.m. I thought about his habit of going to the gym and how it was a convenient excuse that gave him hours of free time and the capacity to return freshly showered. Had I been a fool to be so devoted?

Our sixth wedding anniversary and my ninth week of pregnancy happened over Labour Day weekend. I was reviewing our bank accounts online, a habit I'd newly picked up. I saw charges at a pharmacy in West Hollywood. Isaac told me he was in San Francisco. I texted and called him, asking where he was. He replied by email, rambling on about a sailing lesson at the Berkeley Marina. He said he might not be able to be in touch for a bit. He was caught.

Alone in my apartment, I was sick from betrayal. I called him over and over. When he wouldn't answer, I left terrible messages. I made threats. I was not thinking straight. My head and heart were throbbing and my entire body was consumed in rage. When he finally picked up, he continued to lie to me. So I told him the name of his hotel and he stopped. I demanded to know who he was with. He told me he was with his boyfriend.

Later, I would come to learn that prior to this man, there had been months of experimentation with others, throughout the time we were trying to get pregnant. He would later say he hadn't considered we might actually conceive. This was his excuse for much of his behaviour: he just didn't consider or acknowledge what he was doing, compartmentalizing his lives. That night, as I raged over the phone, the risk of his actions began to sink in. I had to calm down.

Survival kicked in. I owe my life to my baby and how she pushed me to endure that unforgettable evening when my nightmares came true and my monsters were real. I was determined to get help. My doctor was away for a couple of days, but I couldn't imagine sharing this with anyone else. I made an appointment to see her at the first opportunity, on Thursday.

Wednesday, I moved into my new apartment. Like most transitions, it was stressful and demanding. I was nauseated throughout the move and was sick several times. I told myself this meant my baby was still well. I promised her I would love her and protect her from whatever surprises were still in store. I put a bed in the living room that would be mine, and the bedroom would be for the baby. I showed her where her crib would go. The dresser that would be her changing table went against the wall. I put the rabbit on top.

Thursday, I was up early to see my doctor. Feeling sick once again, I threw up in the sewer as I walked down Bay Street. I heard calls from some construction workers perched above in a half-built apartment building. They thought I was drunk. I assured my baby I'd teach her how to ignore men like that.

My doctor was sympathetic when I told her what I'd discovered about Isaac. She had been his doctor as well and, of course, gave no indication if she knew. She ordered the necessary blood work and performed an internal exam. She shared with me her own story of heartbreak and betrayal. Then she gave me a requisition so I could get another ultrasound after my blood work. We agreed that seeing the baby would cheer me up. I promised myself I would finally get a picture. I hadn't requested one at previous appointments because I didn't want to be a bother.

The ultrasound clinic was a few floors below and the wait wasn't long for a walk-in. Soon, I was on the table with cold gel on my stomach. The technician rolled the device over my belly. Her face remained expressionless. She didn't show me the screen and instead excused herself for a few minutes. I enjoyed the last few moments of my pregnancy, alone in that room. I imagined the doctor returning to tell me I was having twins. Something was protecting me, allowing me those last few precious minutes where it did not occur to me that there could be bad news.

A doctor returned with the technician and he sat down next to me. He squirted some more gel on my stomach and rolled the device over me. He stared at the screen. The tech stood behind him. After a few minutes, he quickly pulled away.

He directed his first comment to the tech: "Yep."

She nodded.

And then he said to me, "I'm sorry, there's no heartbeat." He left the room.

I could not move, but I shook from my sobs. The technician wiped my stomach clean and began talking. "It's okay. Go home to your husband. Try again. I'll see you back in a few months." She repeated this refrain as she coaxed me off the table and toward the door. Her hand burned like a hot iron on my back as it pushed me down the hall. She repeated it again: "It's okay. Go home to your husband, I'll see you in a couple of months." She opened the door to my change stall and left.

I dressed and wandered out of the office. Had I been thinking, I would have gone straight to my family doctor. Had the technician been thinking, she would have noticed there was no ring on my finger. Had the clinic called my doctor, she would have helped me. Had they done anything, I may not have ended up on the curb outside the medical building alone, sobbing. My thoughts began to focus on the traffic in front of me. Would I ruin the driver's life if I jumped in front of their car?

Several people stopped and tried to talk to me. I couldn't reply. But when a middle-aged woman wearing a bicycle helmet asked for my phone,

I gave it to her. She had kind eyes. She asked if she could call someone and I pointed to a number. She spoke to Naomi, who was in our office just down the street. Naomi arrived quickly and held me as I cried. She put me in a taxi and gave the driver my parents' address.

As we drove, I told myself my baby was being punished for what I'd done. I thought about how I'd tried to eat as much as I could, but couldn't keep anything down. I thought of all the terrible things I'd said to Isaac when he left me. I thought about how angry I had felt inside when I caught him with his boyfriend. I cried harder, believing I had killed my baby.

I arrived at my childhood home. My mom rushed out the front door and ushered me inside. My dad, aunt, and uncle were there, too. Voices and noises echoed and bounced off the bare walls. My old room had long ago been converted to an office, so I lay down on the couch in the den. Faces around me were blurry through my puffy eyes and tears. I heard them calling out different ways to soothe me. My dad gave me a pill that I swallowed with a cool glass of water handed to me by my mother. I just wanted to sleep, but when I closed my eyes, there was no peace.

My doctor triple checked the death of the baby with blood tests and further ultrasounds. These appointments, although necessary, were agony, as happy, pregnant women and their supportive partners were everywhere. At the ultrasound, I asked for a picture of the baby. I no longer cared about being a bother. I noticed the strange look from the insensitive technician.

I would need to repeat another blood test in six months, but Isaac's infidelity had not given me anything. My body was disease-free, but it had betrayed me and rejected my baby for a reason I'd never know.

I was scared to tell Isaac about the miscarriage. Even after what he'd done, I feared he would disappear, and I couldn't endure another loss. Before I told him, I begged him to be gentle and kind with me. In my grief, I set aside his infidelity for a few weeks. We shared many evenings talking on the phone as I waited for my body to end the pregnancy naturally. We even talked about maybe trying for another child. I couldn't tell anyone I was speaking to him, but I needed his comfort. I felt like a failure as a mother, wife, and woman.

Twenty days later, my body still refused to let my baby go. My mom took me to the hospital so they could take her out. When I woke up, I felt empty and numb. Ironically, the only formal acknowledgement of my loss was from the divorce lawyer I had contacted at my father's request. He sent a beautiful bouquet of flowers. I put them on top of the changing table that would now just be a dresser. I watered and tended to them carefully before they withered away.

I spent the next month grieving intensely, going to therapy several times a week, and discovering more about Isaac's infidelity. The protective fog lifted and I saw that, of course, there was no going back to my husband. It would take months for him to divulge all his betrayals — and there are still things he claimed not to remember. I've accepted that I'll never know it all. In time and without lawyers, we agreed upon a settlement and divorced amicably. We filed the papers at the courthouse together. Years later, we are still in touch. He recently told me he wants children one day. That was hard to hear, maybe because I'm still not recovered enough to be able to say the same.

The insensitivity of the professionals at the ultrasound clinic stayed with me, even months later, so I wrote the staff a letter. When I tell people the date tattooed on my wrist is my baby's due date, I see the uncomfortable looks. I feel less alone when I'm with another childless mother who understands. Most difficult to face are the people who ask me why I am unmarried and don't have children. I get this question often: from the hairdresser, dentist, and store clerks. I give a lot of awkward shrugs and smiles. To friends and family, I am as honest as possible. It's an exercise in trust, which can be risky. It's become easy to discern who has experienced a miscarriage and who likely has not. I once declined a request to plan a baby shower. When I explained that it was difficult for me, the reply was "Still?"

Years later, I see a therapist regularly and have been diagnosed with post-traumatic stress disorder. Weddings, baby showers, and pregnancies are challenging for me. Sometimes I forget myself and chime in about the nuisance of morning sickness with other mothers. If I'm then not able to answer what brand of diapers I use, I feel as though I've been caught trying to sneak into a club. It's as if the experience of pregnancy disappears if you don't give birth. I'm no longer a wife and I don't feel accepted into the circle of motherhood. But I became a mother the moment I became pregnant, as I imagine most mothers whose children are alive might say.

Grieving the loss of the baby has been deeply personal, private, and on-going. On any given day, I know how old she would be. I continue to work on not punishing myself for her death. This and learning to trust are the biggest hurdles that prevent me from trying to conceive again. I try to ig-nore the ticking clock in the background and the many times I've been told my baby's passing was meant to be. Instead, I adopted a kitten. I've enjoyed the freedom I have to travel. I have time for after-work drinks with friends. I take pride in my career and supporting myself independently. I find joy in the small things, such as a new pen or a puppy at the park. I'm enjoying the new role of being an aunt and watching my parents as grandparents. Still living in the same building, I contribute to the care of my now ailing father. It may not be where I expected to be in life, but it is where I am.

The day I married Isaac, wearing my princess dress in the Toronto cas-tle, my dreams came true. Had someone warned me how it was going to end, I wouldn't have believed it. Perhaps that's why we reassure our children their nightmares aren't real. As we grow older, we realize that nightmares often do come true, but we would never want our children to stop trust-ing or taking risks out of fear of getting hurt. We encourage them to keep reaching for the stars, no matter how far away they seem. I now imagine my life like one of the impressionable, recurring dreams from my childhood: sometimes unexpected, but capable of being resolved with love, with sup-port, and by just getting out of bed in the morning.

7

AUDREY

Meaghan Mazurek

A WEDDING DRESS HUNG in my closet. The venue was booked and the food had been tasted. I knew the sound 100 invitations made when they hit the bottom of a red post box.

My fiancé, Eric, had left Canada to teach in Taiwan for a semester and was getting ready to come home soon. Back in Guelph, I prepared my students for their June exams. Eric and I had spent the last five months talking on Skype about our upcoming wedding and the life we wanted to build together. We dreamed of buying a big old house and filling it with tiny humans who looked a bit like both of us.

A week before his flight home, Eric called me. I was sitting in my office at work, marking final projects. I grabbed my phone and went outside to sit in the sunshine.

"Hey." His voice sounded strange.

"What's wrong?" I asked.

"Nothing."

"No, seriously, what is it?" I pressed.

"I'm sorry," he said. "I don't really know how to say this.... I don't think I can marry you."

His words made the $900 dress hanging in my closet utterly useless. I cried for days, big, ugly sobs.

A week after Eric called off our wedding, I turned 29 and my uterus quivered in terror. I wanted a big family and until recently, having kids had been right around the corner. Now I would have to date. Dating was bullshit. Not having to date again was one of the awesome things about getting married.

I cried some more. For months I moped around, wrote sad songs, and called everyone I knew, trying to fill my house with noise. I travelled to new countries, alone, to make new memories that didn't include Eric.

To my great luck, there were lovely humans not yet claimed. Seven months after that dreadful day with Eric, I found one. I met Matt.

Matt and I leaped into a big new love. We'd spent our 20s in drawn-out relationships with people our families disliked. We now knew what we wanted in a partner. We moved in after two months of dating. Five months after that, we rudely monopolized our friends and family on their last summer long weekend for our wedding.

When you know, you know.

After the wedding, I settled into a new school year. At night, I took yoga classes and constantly read. I was always picking up new books I'd put on hold at the library. Matt worked as an engineer, and in the evenings he took a commercial photography course. We both wanted kids and knew our free time would soon be in short supply, so we enjoyed every minute of it while we still could.

We started trying to have a baby immediately after we were married, happily counting the months on our fingers.

"If it works this time, I'll be pregnant in July!" I said.

But after three months of trying, all I had was a nasty, recurrent urinary tract infection. By the fifth month, the world seemed full of babies and pregnant people, and strangely I somehow still wasn't one of them. All those years of fear-fuelled birth control for nothing.

After six months, Matt lied to his doctor about how long we'd been trying, and the doctor ordered some tests. Soon after, he called us with the results. Matt's sperm count was low, but we had no sense of scale. How low? Was it even possible for us to get pregnant naturally?

"A specialist will call you," the doctor told Matt.

That office called Matt with an appointment, but it wasn't for another three months. Three months felt like three years. I needed more information. While we waited, I started tracking my temperature, trying to pinpoint ovulation, but my numbers varied wildly and the process only stressed me out more.

When Matt's appointment finally arrived, we battled the traffic into Toronto, parked our Rabbit, and put an outrageous amount of money into the parking machine. After two hours of boredom in a bland waiting room, we found out Matt's low was *really* low. His sample had about a million sperm, compared to the 20 to 40 million the doctor expected to see. And the sperm that did exist had bad motility.

"They're deformed," the doctor said. "They probably swim in circles." He gave us a few options. Surgery for Matt had a 50-50 chance of improving his sperm count. And if that didn't work, in vitro fertilization (IVF) with intracytoplasmic sperm injection (ICSI) was our next best option.

IVF: the big guns. I knew vaguely of it — a friend had IVF twins — but if I'd known more about what it entailed, I would have been alarmed. Instead, I was just surprised and sad we were unlikely to conceive on our own.

I was grateful for a diagnosis, though. It helped to have a name for this thing and the specific steps required in order for us to move forward. Friends had dealt with the uncertainty and frustration of being designated with "unexplained infertility," as though that could ever really be a diagnosis.

We opened up to some friends and family, as I refused to go through this alone. We received much love and support, but also heard many frustrating comments. My mother, who lovingly talked me down every time I called her crying, often asked if we'd looked into using Clomid, a drug meant to improve ovulation. Others asked us this, too. Clomid was the infertility drug most people seemed to have heard of. In fact, our specialist had put Matt on the drug. Few people know that it can also help men with sperm issues by increasing testosterone levels. The prescription alarmed our pharmacist.

"Are you sure this is right?" he asked. "I've never heard of Clomid being used for" — he lowered his voice further — "a man?" The prescription was right, but unfortunately it didn't help Matt's count.

When I opened up to anyone new, they always assumed the issue was with me. Even after I told people we'd had a clear diagnosis of male factor infertility, I was still asked if I'd been tested for issues.

Another common response to disclosing our infertility was the advice to "just adopt," which seemed to totally ignore the reality of adoption in Canada. In most jurisdictions in Canada, it's an arduous process that can take many years.

This brand of advice seemed to completely minimize my need to experience pregnancy. It felt impossible to explain how essential pregnancy was to me. I didn't just want a child; I wanted to carry that child and give birth to it. It was less about having a baby to share my genes and more about a deep need I'd felt for many years to have this experience.

One year for Halloween, when I was maybe 9 or 10, I dressed up as a frazzled pregnant woman. I had wild hair and I wore a housecoat and a stuffed backpack on my front. It seems like an odd choice now, but even then my uterus ached for the experience of pregnancy, and that ache hadn't let up since.

I couldn't always describe to people what it was about pregnancy that I needed so badly, but at some point I realized I didn't have to explain it to others. The need to experience pregnancy and childbirth felt as real as to me the need for food and water. We had been trying for only a year, but I couldn't seem to go more than four minutes without remembering that we hadn't been able to get pregnant.

For Matt, that thought was always followed by the word *yet*: "We haven't gotten pregnant yet." His optimism kept me going but also made me angry.

"Why aren't you worried?" I asked him repeatedly. "What if none of this works?

"It'll work," he said, again and again, his voice calm. "I know it will."

"But you can't know that. No one is promising us anything."

"We'll find a way to get pregnant. I know we will."

We soon gave Matt's optimism a name: Audrey. Matt had fond memories of his grandmother Audrey and hoped that someday a daughter of ours might share her name. The word became shorthand for a happy future. "Just remember Audrey," he often told me.

We had this conversation over and over. I would often shit on his optimism because I couldn't understand how it came so effortlessly to him. But I also needed it, badly. I couldn't have lived through those years without his faith.

Matt's surgery went well enough. We got him home safely and his recovery went smoothly. The surgery didn't change his sperm count, though, which meant the next step was going to be IVF.

I have a lifelong phobia of needles, and IVF is essentially just a whole bunch of needles: blood draws, drug injections, and one massive needle for the egg retrieval, with a ton of internal ultrasounds thrown in for funsies. Living an hour away from the nearest fertility clinic made it even more challenging to get there every other morning for many weeks at a time.

It took the grinding reality of IVF — clinic visits, blood draws, internal ultrasounds — for me to realize what the sperm specialist had really been saying to us that day: Matt, your sperm don't swim. Meaghan, you will receive all the medical treatment for Matt's health issue. Matt will continue to be your loving support person. He will offer a steady hand for injections, and one day soon, he will need to jizz into a cup. The specialist didn't warn me that I might feel angry about my healthy body being poked and prodded while Matt stood on the sidelines.

Also, no one warned us about the embryo-update phone calls. After the IVF egg retrieval and the fertilization of those eggs with Matt's sperm, the lab called us every morning to tell us how many had survived the night. We started with a very satisfying 11.

Day 5 was a snow day and I was out shovelling when we got the call. There were two: two embryos left. Over $10,000 and what felt like a million needles, and we had only two. Two chances for a baby.

Our doctor argued for single embryo transfers. Twelve days after the first embryo transfer we drove to the clinic to get a blood test. Then I went to work, trying, and mostly failing, to think about other things. Just after lunch I got the phone call. The nurse's voice was low. "I'm sorry; the test was negative."

We were not pregnant.

I had to leave the office to go teach fourth period with bloodshot eyes. My students knew something was up and treaded gently with me.

On the drive home from work, I cried some more. One chance left. We had one more chance to avoid doing IVF again.

The second call came two months later. I sat in our backyard while Matt answered the phone. Despite the warm sun, I shivered wildly. I heard the screen door open. I looked up and saw Matt's face and I knew it didn't work.

After the second transfer failed, we sat down to talk with our doctor. Through our devastation came a determination to try again, just not IVF. Pushing forward using Matt's sperm didn't feel right to either of us. We asked our doctor about doing an unmedicated round of artificial intrauterine insemination (IUI) with donor sperm. He was surprised by our request.

"Why not try IVF again?" he asked, his framed degrees scattered on the wall behind his head.

There were many reasons why we didn't want to do IVF again. We both wanted to try something less invasive, since no one could tell us if Matt's sperm quality had contributed to the loss of so many embryos. Matt was uncomfortable with the IVF-level of intervention and worried a child conceived from his scanty, malformed sperm might have health issues. Neither of us had been able to forget the day another sperm specialist warned us Matt's genetic male children might experience infertility themselves.

Matt was also weirdly okay with using a donor. He didn't have any angst around it. Instead, the idea gave him a sense of relief. If we proceeded with a donor, he wouldn't have to worry about the toll IVF took on my body or our marriage.

We had already started looking at donor catalogues, which was basically like online dating. Almost all the sperm donors were American. In Canada, it's illegal to pay for sperm donation, so there aren't many Canadian sperm bank options. After a few hours of searching, we'd found a donor with blue eyes and dark hair, like Matt. His essay was well written and his favourite book was the same as ours.

After a long discussion, our doctor agreed to our plan, and just like that we were back on the horse.

"There's nothing wrong with you," Matt said to me on one of our nightly walks in a nearby park. "If we use donor sperm, this will definitely work."

After the invasiveness of IVF, it was hard to remember that there was nothing wrong with me. Matt was right — it did work. We got pregnant on our first donor IUI, without any medication. When we got the phone call from the fertility clinic, I didn't believe the nurse who gave us the good news.

"Are you sure?" I asked.

"For sure. You are pregnant."

"How pregnant?"

She laughed. "Very pregnant."

I felt like I had finally joined an exclusive club. I drove an hour and a half to Markham, where my parents were visiting relatives, so I could see the look on my mom's face when I told her.

There was nothing wrong with me, but there is random bad luck that may apply to anyone who becomes pregnant.

At the six-week ultrasound, the technician didn't see anything. She handed us a picture of an empty sac floating in space.

"Don't worry," she said. "It could just be too early."

I wasn't sure how that was possible, given that they knew the exact day viable sperm had been placed in my cervix. I also wasn't sure why she thought I'd want an ultrasound picture of nothing.

Matt and I spent a week of hell, in limbo, until a second ultrasound confirmed there was no baby. We fell apart, together. It seemed too cruel, given the two years it had taken us to become pregnant.

A few days later the bleeding started, and with it came cramps like I had never experienced before. Those cramps made me wonder, unironically, if I would even be able to handle the pain of labour if we got pregnant again. I lay on my floor, bent in half, my heart and body aching.

All the platitudes people offered when they heard about our loss just didn't seem appropriate. It had taken two years to get pregnant; there was no guarantee we'd get another chance.

When Matt had been diagnosed with male factor infertility, I searched everywhere for books that might help me understand our situation. Now that our circumstances had changed, I did a new Google search: *loss after infertility.* I found one slim, self-published book and ordered it immediately. When it arrived in the mail, I devoured every word. Someone out there knew what it felt like to experience miscarriage after tough years of infertility. I wanted to hug this woman for making me feel less alone.

Matt's aunt, when she heard about our miscarriage, said, "If people knew how many pregnancies end in miscarriage, they wouldn't be so surprised when they happen."

But I didn't know that. I didn't know how many of my friends and acquaintances had suffered miscarriages until much, much later. Too many women in my life suffered in silence.

My heart and body healed, and too soon, I insisted we go back to the clinic to start trying again. We did six IUIs in seven months, only taking a break for the Christmas office closure. Cycle after cycle, we went from failure to trying again far too quickly.

We found a few ways to make the visits to the clinic more tolerable. After difficult appointments, we rewarded ourselves with lattes from the shop a block away from the clinic. We also started ignoring some of the clinic's procedures, which not all the staff appreciated.

"Don't forget, you need to call on Day One, and come in on Day Three," the ultrasound tech said, snapping off her blue latex gloves. "Every single cycle."

I smiled and nodded, while inside my head a child sulked. *The doctor said it was okay to come in on Day 11*, I thought. But I kept my mouth shut. Out loud, I would sound too much like a child wheedling to one parent that the other parent let us stay up late to watch TV.

When the nurse left the room, I whined out loud to Matt. "It's so dumb. We've done this a million times. We know I ovulate on Day Sixteen. Why would we come in on Day Three? What would those tests tell them? Nothing."

"I know," he said, "but we have to play nice."

Despite fighting hard for fewer visits each cycle, the pace of our back-to-back cycles made me miserable. Looking back, I can't imagine why we didn't take more breaks, but at the time it felt essential to plough on. I believed pregnancy could be just around the corner if we only had enough stamina to continue. We also knew we could get pregnant without medication, so every time the doctor insisted we try a medicated IUI cycle, we reminded him I had gotten pregnant without medication and believed I could again. We were just waiting for that next big fat positive.

It became harder and harder to believe that nothing was wrong with me. Why wasn't I getting pregnant again? Matt did his best to keep my faith alive, but I spent a lot of time feeling angry at him because he seemed so unscathed by infertility. He wasn't, of course, but I couldn't see past my own pain. He didn't seem worried or miserable like I was. I thought maybe that was because he knew he could live without kids. I didn't know if I could. He felt like a life with just the two of us could be happy. I hated myself a little because I knew I couldn't say the same.

I spent my years of infertility in absolute terror. *What if none of this works?* This thought intruded on my life every day for five years. Fear ruined birthdays and Christmases and every trip we took hoping it would be the last one without kids. I would have paid large sums of money to experience a single day without fear; I would have given up a piano-playing finger for that feeling.

On our eighth try, we got another positive test. This time I told fewer people and felt only cautiously optimistic. Still, with every day that passed, I believed a little bit more that it was finally our turn. At the first ultrasound, though, our worst fears were confirmed. The tech did the scan silently, and when it came time to get Matt so he could see the screen, she just said we should call our doctor.

"No," I told her. Our doctor was on holiday. There was no way I was leaving without more information. "Please tell us something."

"There's nothing to see yet," she told us. I fell apart, sobbing, on the hospital floor. She ran to get Matt.

Somehow, after three years of trying and two positive pregnancy tests, we still didn't have a baby. I hated my life to a degree I would never have believed possible. It felt like nothing was up to us. Every September I returned to teaching, despite my frail optimism that *this* would be our year.

We slogged through the 30-hour training course required to become eligible for public adoption, and a kind social worker did our home study. We hoped it might help us feel like there were different ways we could grow our family. Going through the process only increased my anger exponentially. Filling out the range of acceptance forms felt impossible. How could I possibly decide what physical and mental disabilities I was open to accepting in an adoptive child? How could *anyone* make these kinds of decisions? Agreeing to almost any of the disabilities seemed to require a strength I just didn't have. Infertility treatments and miscarriage had worn me down, made me someone I didn't like. I had lost my happy nature and my smile. Even a simple question from a stranger like "How are you?" had the power to undo me, bring tears to my eyes, and make me run off.

Something had to change. For years I believed we would be happy as soon as we got and stayed pregnant. But now we still weren't pregnant and we weren't willing to give up either. How long was I willing to live unhappily?

The idea of a long break planted itself like a seed in my head. In the past it hadn't felt possible, but now it felt necessary. That didn't mean I was sure I could do it, though. Can you stop trying once you've started? Can you really corral that horse back in the barn, at least temporarily? The more I thought about it, the stronger I felt about taking a break. Here was something I could choose. The idea of a break from trying expanded into a break from work, too. I needed space and time to do something different. I could teach part-time and write for a few hours a day. I'd written a newspaper column when I was in university, and the deadlines had fuelled me and forced me to sit down to do something I loved.

The idea of a leave became reality. The important people in our life of infertility — my mom, our kind and concerned doctor, my close friends — all encouraged us to give ourselves some breathing space.

I spent a lot of my leave writing. I also napped often, like our cat, and learned how to make a mean bolognese sauce from an Italian mama. An energy healer, a job title that made me giggle even as I handed over hard-earned cash, helped me move through some of the fear that had kept me stuck. I volunteered to cook at a shelter for teenage girls, which meant I spent two hours a week teaching them how to cook from simple recipes instead of ruminating on my own sadness.

I learned how to meditate, sitting 10 minutes each day. Most times it felt like I failed to achieve any sort of calm state or clear mind. But as the days added up to weeks and months, sitting helped me have more moments of feeling neutral instead of feeling crappy. My second meditation teacher told me it was okay to meditate comfortably while sitting on a chair, and I haven't stopped meditating since receiving that lesson.

With some distance from the life of trying, I could see that taking a break from treatments, the clinic, and work was the best decision we'd made in our years of infertility. I felt empowered.

Stepping back also helped me see the other choices we'd made more clearly. I saw how foolish the back-to-back IUIs had been. Every cycle had ended the same day the next began, leaving me no room to breathe, let alone to grieve. We'd gone straight from the devastating failure of IVF to a donor IUI that ended in miscarriage. And after eight more tries and another pregnancy loss, I had jumped right back in. My single-minded determination to just keep going until something worked blinded me to the damage I was doing to myself and to my marriage.

Matt had always advocated for breaks, but it had always felt impossible. Now, breaks between cycles felt absolutely necessary. I had found a way to like my life again, and I no longer wanted to give that away in the mindless pursuit of kids.

After our break from trying, we tried four IUIs, but the failures didn't undo me the way they had in the past. It would be another year before we found out an acquaintance was donating to one of the few Canadian sperm banks. He was willing to help us, if we wanted.

We did. After spending almost $30,000 trying to have a child, we tried home inseminations with our acquaintance's sperm, which was basically free. When people asked how we did it, I explained that we used the turkey baster method, though in reality we used a sample cup and a needleless syringe. It seemed impossible that a process so simple could work, but on the second try, it did.

Years of infertility and multiple miscarriages meant I worried my way through the first five months of pregnancy. Because of our previous losses, we had a lot of ultrasounds early in this pregnancy, and I began each one by asking the technician if the baby was still alive. Seeing our baby's tiny feet and hands and heart moving on the screen gave me a few hours, sometimes even days, free of anxiety. When my worries returned, I often found myself making a mental list of all the people who knew we were pregnant. These were the people I'd have to email when everything went wrong.

Nothing went wrong, though, and the second half of my pregnancy was much better. Once I could feel the baby's constant movements, my fear decreased significantly and I finally let myself get excited.

Our daughter was born October 30, 2016, in our bedroom, with a team of midwives and Matt sitting behind me. When one of the women placed this brand-new baby in our arms, I felt a surge of relief.

We could stop trying. Audrey had arrived.

8

BORN OUT OF STILLNESS

Carine Blin

Associations and sensations are flooding in and being held by the fluid.
— Carole Maso, *Mother and Child*

FOR THE MOST PART, I've stopped wondering when Jacob floated into stillness, suspended in amniotic fluid. The feelings of guilt subsided long ago, but the fact that I will never be able to pinpoint the moment when he died still lingers in my mind.

How did he get tangled up? Was he doing flip turns or somersaults? At 39 weeks' gestation, there isn't much space to move around.

The doctors told us it was a cord accident and we never doubted their conclusion. The lesions on Jacob's neck seemed evidence enough. Perhaps he'd been awakening to the pleasant sensation of stretching his limbs, tumbling in slow motion like an astronaut tethered on a spacewalk. Maybe he got carried away in a dreamy reverie and I forgot to warn him about getting too wrapped up in his lifeline. At least this is the story I tell myself.

In the narrative that spins inside my head, he was always a swimmer, like his siblings. The two who came before him and the one after. They carry the marker of their father's genetic signature: water babies, all of them. Comfortable when submersed, giddily frolicking naked in the rain, crouching on a wave, or skimming the surface of a lap pool. They swim end-to-end lengths of front crawl to the rhythm of a heartbeat and the sound of their steady breath, bubbling underwater. Our four children were aquatic creatures from the moment of their conception.

Jacob's death in utero was confirmed by an ultrasound. I knew it was unusual for our midwife to request an ultrasound mere days before his due date. At our scheduled Friday appointment, she expressed some concern about his growth since the last time we had met. There didn't appear to be any immediate cause for alarm. The first available appointment for the scan was on the following Monday.

For three days, I tried to carry on as if nothing had changed. I'm not sure I was conscious of the unsettling thoughts floating inside my head. I was more focused on telling myself there was nothing to worry about and keeping myself distracted.

On the Friday morning, Jacob's heartbeat had been normal. That meant he was okay. I went to see a movie in the middle of the day to pass the time, but I should have known better than to choose a Stanley Kubrick film that left me agitated, sitting alone in the darkness. The next morning, I attended a stretching class for pregnant moms. There was a moment during the class when I rolled over on the mat and felt my baby drop from one side to the other. Something about the way everything shifted felt unfamiliar. I simply attributed it to the difficulty I was having moving gracefully in the final week of pregnancy. I never asked anyone to explain what this could have meant. It wouldn't have changed a thing. It's just a detail that insists on remaining in the story.

On the Saturday afternoon, I took my five-year-old son to a salon for his first professional haircut. We took a photo from the newspaper because he wanted to come out looking like Mike Johnson of the Toronto Maple Leafs. I was distracted on the way home, thinking about my upcoming appointment. That night, during dinner with friends, I lay down on their living room couch to rest, waiting to feel the faint pressure of Jacob kicking inside of me. Sunday is a complete blank. I don't recall anything about it.

Many details surrounding the circumstances of Jacob's birth have since eluded me, but the memory of the last ultrasound is crystal clear. The moment the technician looked at me and then backed herself out of the ultrasound room, I knew for certain Jacob was dead. A voice inside told me to stay quiet, to lie still, to let the story unfold. I stared at the fluorescent light above and at the back of the black monitor, took in the size of the room, and imagined voices on the other side of the door discussing how high-frequency sound waves shatter dreams on some workdays. The second hand was banging inside my head and circling the face of the clock. His due date was still one week away.

Time is erratic when you are filled with dread about what is going to happen next. When you are lying on a hospital cot waiting for someone to walk you down the hall to meet the doctor in charge so he can tell you straight out that your baby has no heartbeat. Time can disappear when you fix your eyes on the white lab coat ahead of you on your way to receive this news. It can stop entirely when you listen in disbelief to what the doctor has to say to you. The physician is old enough to look, and sound, authoritative. He is dressed like a professional. His tone is measured. He's practised in the language of scientific evidence, whether the news is good or bad. He knows how to make the message clear and concise so there will be no misunderstanding. He needs to look you in the eyes so you can absorb the gravity of what he has to say. You already know anyway. You've had 10 minutes to think on it, and you'll have the rest of your life to pull apart each strand of this unwelcome story, rework it, and pattern a narrative to give it some sense.

I remember listening carefully to the words being spoken at me and trying to grasp the meaning. I understood that I did not have to deliver the baby right away. The physician said, "There is no rush. No danger in waiting. Go home and talk it over with your husband. Take your time."

It seemed obvious there was no longer any danger to my baby, and it never occurred to me to even consider any risk to myself. All I could think about was the fact that I had failed to protect my baby in my womb. I wanted to get him out of there as soon as possible, and I couldn't come up with a single reason to prolong the distressing situation I was in. The thought of going to bed knowing my baby had died was so disquieting, the more I dwelled on it the quicker I wanted to go home, pack my things, and head off to our local hospital so I could give birth.

The day I lost Jacob and the days and weeks and months following were filled with sadness and yearning. I felt disconnected and angry and disappointed in my interactions with other people. But I also appreciated compassionate words and gestures that stopped me from feeling alone in my sorrow. The first time this happened, I was being escorted out of the hospital the day of the ultrasound. The technician who helped me find a taxi was not the one who had performed the ultrasound, because that staff person was too unnerved with how her day had begun. I don't blame her. The second technician was more at ease in the presence of loss. She gave me a kind look, one that touched gently on my aching heart. She took my arm in hers to steady me a little. The soft pressure of her hand felt like the sprinkling of stars. On the way to the elevator we passed the same parents who had been waiting in line when I arrived earlier that morning. They were still there, chatting and smiling, anticipating a quick peek at baby in vitro before taking home a paper image from the sonogram to stick on the fridge door. Maybe they would even ask to know the gender because that seemed to be a matter of importance to them.

I glanced at the pregnant women as I walked past and I thought about the bond between mother and unborn child. Like an unyielding force pulling at the reaches of a private universe. From the instant my first baby stirred as a tiny sparkle in a secret part of my womb, I was smitten with love. I drew him close and cradled him inside the darkness while I carried on with my routines. The sonograms these women now lined up for barely captured the edges of a two-dimensional image. They couldn't render the emotional resonance of a mother's deep longing to hold her baby in her arms, to look after him.

My third pregnancy, with Jacob, was a blissful period up until that last visit with my midwife. There's a photo of me tucked into an album. In it, I am lying on a beach in Mexico, beside my husband, sometime during the second trimester, my arms and legs wrapped around him, basking in a moment of tenderness. I remember embracing the fullness of my pregnant body, attuned to the stirrings of my baby and the physical changes and hormonal fluctuations in me. The thought that something could go wrong never entered my mind. I didn't know that 7 out of every 1,000 births in Canada end in stillbirth. It's hard to imagine you will be that statistic when the sky looks clear from your soft place in the sand and the forecast is sunny for the foreseeable future.

I drifted through those happy months with a lightness of being, glancing down at the waterline where sand and ripple mix to toss up the occasional piece of glistening sea glass. I couldn't wait to submerse myself in the choppy waters of childbirth, wrestling with my body to deliver my baby safely onto solid ground where he would feel the air on his skin and would fill his lungs for the first time.

By the time Jacob was born, I had already experienced labour twice, once in hospital and once at home. Giving birth had felt natural and instinctual, even though it was intense and painful. I drew air in big gulps as the contractions intensified. I was seized with the cramping, trying to breathe steadily, waiting for some relief and steeling myself for the next round. It was exhilarating and exhausting. I was tapping into a deep store of energy, carried by a long-awaited promise, concentration derailed by violent physical upheaval, a kind of womb eruption ending with a feeling of euphoria as I cradled my newborn in my arms and then handed our baby to his adoring father.

The night Jacob was born, I laboured in the same hospital bed where I had delivered his older brother five years earlier. The birthing room was reserved for natural childbirths and, presumably, for miscarriages and stillbirths. The space was a nondescript beige. There were two standard-issue hospital-room chairs beside the bed, a floral pink and beige bedspread, a small side table, a bare floor, a white ceiling with fluorescent lighting, four solid walls, and a private bathroom. There is nothing private about giving birth, so being steps away from my own bathroom while I was between contractions mattered more than the drab details of the room. In retrospect, none of that really mattered. All I wanted was for my son to be born alive and healthy.

The doctor who had delivered my first-born years earlier in that same drab birthing room was a francophile. My French name prompted him to engage in a conversation about Paris, in French, so he was somewhat distracted when he finally realized the baby's head was crowning. That precipitated a flurry of activity. He scrambled to pull on a pair of blue latex gloves while calling down the hall for the nurses to leave their staff meeting so they could help him catch the baby in time. I would have preferred to deliver at home in the care of a midwife, but at the time midwifery wasn't widely practised in Ontario, and given that I had a short and uncomplicated delivery, this first birth was as perfect as I could have wished for.

My daughter was born 19 months later, at home and in the care of a wise, silver-haired midwife who tiptoed around the bedroom in her flowing robes, whispering encouragement, quietly exuding grace and confidence. Her smiling eyes had inspected a thousand newborns and concluded, every time, that catching a baby was just an ordinary miracle under the light of a double rainbow. When the birth is straightforward and followed by a celebratory glass of bubbly and the chance to slip into a warm bath with your new baby snuggled against you, everything seems right with the world.

My first two babies chose the timing of their arrival. With Jacob, I had to choose. Though I was knotted up inside, I clung to my vision of a natural childbirth, my own nine-months pregnant body in tune with a rhythm that was bred in the bone. I told myself his birth was going to be straightforward. I knew what to do. This still seemed in my control on a day when everything else had turned out so wrong.

When my husband and I arrived at the hospital where Jacob was born late on the day of the ultrasound, I tried to steady my gaze as I moved through the heavy glass doors, toward a large elevator, and then up to the maternity ward, where nursing staff were waiting to check us in. I could tell from their faces and their flat tones that they had been forewarned. It was a quiet night on the ward, but I imagined labouring women on either side of the hallway, separated from us by a curtain in their small stalls. I thought about those mothers seeing their babies' eyes open and hearing their babies' voices mark day one with that unmistakable cry of a newborn.

The induction was precipitated with a round of pills. People around me seemed kind but intent on offering me more drugs so I could blur my way through this mess, as if looking through a windshield in the teeming rain. I preferred a clear view of things, so I concentrated on finding my focus, breathing in the compassion in the room, and arriving at our meeting place — my destiny — with Jacob. I drank black tea and waited in silence.

It's hard to consider the practical details when you contemplate the idea of going into labour with a baby who is dead inside you. It's hard to make decisions or filter out what is being said around you so you can listen to your own intuitive inner voice. I think we agreed not to send for our two young children to meet Jacob because we didn't want to scare them. We didn't invite anyone else into our birthing room. Perhaps we were too frightened ourselves, or maybe it was something else. It felt like the right thing to do, but we regretted it later and all we could tell ourselves, and our children, was that we did the best we could in that moment.

We never thought to bring a camera to the hospital. One of the nurses on duty offered to take a photo with a Polaroid camera. She assured us it was a good idea, that we would treasure it later, that we would have something to remember him by. At the time, it seemed inconsequential. Later we realized it was the only likeness of our child. The only photographic evidence of his brief life with us, those few hours we huddled together inside hospital walls while he lay swaddled in blankets knit by kind-hearted women with time on their hands. During a period in our grief when it felt as though no one understood the extent of our pain, that photo was material proof of Jacob's existence. Only those of us in the room the night he was born — and the people who handled his body after we left him — ever saw his face. The framed photo remained on the kitchen counter for many years as a way to keep him present not only for ourselves, but also for anyone who happened to walk by.

Infant loss is often referred to as a disenfranchised loss, one that is not openly acknowledged or publicly mourned the same way our society mourns the loss of a child or adult they have known. When there are no shared stories or memories and few reminders, the path to healing is particularly long and difficult and lonely. It is one of the heavy burdens bereaved parents suffer when their child is born still.

Before the days of digital photos, Polaroid prints offered an instant likeness on a square sheet of glossy paper with white borders, but the quality was poor and the image washed out over time. Someone suggested we get the photo of Jacob retouched and printed on high quality paper. We agreed to have it enhanced because Jacob's skin was discoloured and looked withered. I thought about how hard it would be to share that image with anyone. I'm not sure anymore that it was the right thing to do, because the photo doesn't bear any real semblance. Nowadays it is nearly impossible to conjure up the details of his facial features, his little hands, or the weight of him in my arms. My memory has faded like the original photo.

When we gave our permission to release Jacob to the doctors early the next morning, the nurses and the two midwives who attended the birth made sure we were given Jacob's footprints and handprints in blue ink on a thick piece of card stock. They also left us with a lock of his dark hair in a little ceramic box, the yellow knitted blanket they had wrapped him in, and the tiny hat he had worn. We left the hospital empty handed except for some official paperwork and these few mementos. Walking out the door without him was heartbreaking, but we didn't think to take him home, nor was that an option we were asked to consider. We were spent. Even staying at the hospital any longer that morning seemed pointless. We signed some forms authorizing an autopsy to confirm the cause of death — we must have been compelled to know "for sure" — and then we walked away and tried not to think about where they were taking him or what would happen to him next.

It took a long time — much longer than anyone anticipates — to stop dwelling on the anguish of leaving the hospital without my baby. I felt gutted. I knew our children would be waiting for us, but I wasn't ready to go home and neither was my husband. Instead, we headed to a hotel downtown and asked for a room, but the woman at the front desk said she had nothing available, so we stayed a while quietly sobbing in the breakfast room at a small table near the window overlooking the lake, as far away as possible from where hotel guests were reading the morning news. A waitress smiled kindly at us and brought coffee and tissues, and when it seemed we had been there long enough, we headed home, gathered our children around the sandbox in the backyard, and tried to explain that something very sad had happened. Jacob was never coming home. We left it to our sister to face their bewilderment as we went to hide under the sheets upstairs.

Then there was a week of forward movement and activity. I made arrangements to collect Jacob's ashes, a task that precipitated a rare moment of black humour. When the funeral director arrived at our front door in the pouring rain, he handed me a small box with Jacob's name misspelled on the label. Then he tried to sell me on the benefits of prepaid burial plots. It felt good to find the humour in this surreal conversation and, later, to feel energized enough to organize a small memorial ceremony with our immediate family and our closest friends and to plan an escape for a weekend up north alone with my husband so we could mourn our loss together. But there everything stopped. Surrounded by nature in a tranquil setting, we went through the motions of walking, eating, and sleeping. Not even the voices of the forest could stir our senses because we were consumed with our own sadness and anger and self-pity.

In the midst of that pain, I also felt stirrings of a bittersweet story in the making. From the start, the memory of Jacob's birthing was tender. He had come to us in the middle of a clear summer night. He came gently. Slipped into the world without a whimper. Into a room that stayed completely and utterly silent. I don't know the colour of his eyes but his little limp body was perfect. He lay cuddled in his father's arms for a long time while I looked on, emptied and disoriented. We declined, then accepted, an invitation from the minister on call to join us, because we were utterly lost. This spiritual man came to assure us that there was still grace and love in the world, even in the midst of our grief. He made us laugh, even in those terrible hours, and allowed us both to cry our tears and hold each other desperately until the sun came up and there seemed nothing more to do but walk away.

Once you lose a child, you remain a bereaved parent for the rest of your life. But what you cannot see plainly when grief is raw and constant is the power of loss and suffering to magnify love. I discovered this when I attended a support group and, later, when I began volunteering to help other parents who had experienced infant loss. But in the wake of my loss, it was all I could do to see daylight. I remember a long period after Jacob died as a black void in my life, when I retreated behind the closed curtains of my living room, cloistered in my grief books and my solitariness. I was angry that others did not seem to comprehend the all-consuming love of a mother who dreams of her baby long before the moment of conception and who wraps the child inside her for nine months, the two of them entangled in mutual contemplation. I was vulnerable to comments that burned: "You're still young." "You can have another one." "It was meant to be." "Worse things can happen." "You are lucky — think of the two you have at home." All true. All hurtful. All innocently intended to distract from the conversation about grief.

In Western culture, we are reluctant to talk about death because it makes us uncomfortable, even squirmy. When my baby died, people around me found it impossible to know what to say or how to react. I wanted them to listen, but I didn't quite know how to tell them what I needed. When I felt brave enough to go out in the world, I wanted some visible sign, some article of clothing or symbol I could wear to let everyone know I was bereaved. I wanted people to acknowledge him, but it seemed hard for some to mention Jacob's name. I think they were worried about triggering my grief, but I wanted to tell them that grief was my constant companion, even if it was thinly veiled beneath an effort to appear fine. That hearing Jacob's name on their lips was like waking up to the sound of the last songbird to head south. I was never quite sure when that lyrical call would return, but I was predisposed to wish for its musical tone, even in the dead of winter.

When I lost Jacob, I was handed a gift. I didn't believe it when a friend told me something precious could come from so much pain, but she was right. For a long time, I needed to stay under the surface, fill my lungs with longing and sadness, fold into myself, and sit with my grief. I also needed to release it by writing, crying — alone and sometimes in public — and talking about it. I was doubly blessed with friends and family members who were patient with me, who indulged my sadness so I could discover the antidote to my suffering through love. I already had an inkling about the infinite store of love a mother could summon for her children; I knew the intoxicating scent and taste of romantic love; I felt the enduring love of next of kin; and now I began to experience a connection in the presence of another person's grief that was filled with loving kindness and compassion. Learning to be in that moment without judgment and without the need to solve anything was restorative and profoundly healing. In the presence of loss, I came to experience an uncommon fullness of life, a counterpoint to the shadows, a wellspring of gratitude.

The first time I connected this way with a complete stranger was when I met with a mother whose son was also born still in midsummer. We sat face to face in a coffee shop, and I lost track of time as she disclosed the details of her story to me. We talked about our babies, found common ground in other aspects of our lives, and became friends in an instant. She cried and she smiled and we laughed together. I could see this release of emotion was cathartic and healing for her. For me. Outside, monarchs were leaving their northern breeding grounds, returning to Mexico on winds and spiralling columns of warm air. She and I were part of our own shimmering cluster, looking for a place of refuge. I was being swept in the right direction, volunteering with a local charitable organization that matched volunteers with people whose stories of loss were similar. I was busy finding meaning by caring for others. Participating in an infant-loss support group and attending volunteer training exposed me to many different stories and helped me step outside the corners of my own experience. But this one-to-one meeting with a grieving mother was the first time I experienced compassion as a flood of emotion that transported me to a place of peace. It was a moment of awakening.

Feeling compassion because we identify with someone's pain is not the same as truly understanding someone's experience. Bereavement literature teaches us that each person's grief is unique, but when we recognize similarities between our own story and someone else's, it's tempting to think we understand. I don't think we can ever come close to knowing what the other person is going through. In fact, I remember recoiling any time someone said to me, "I understand."

Even when our losses look comparable on the surface, there are many aspects to our stories that make them singularly our own. There is nothing to be gained by comparing our losses and everything to be gained by listening to the storyteller. In all my encounters with bereaved parents, the willingness to listen and bear witness has always struck me as the most sincere and loving way to act as a support. By doing so, we help prepare the ground for each person's story to take flight. That is the best we can do.

I'm glad I was patient with myself. There were days when the heat was unbearable. I could hardly lift myself out of my lethargy to take care of my two young children, but being in their presence made me smile. I sensed that if I just let the anguish and pain wash over me without resisting, it would eventually run its course. There were beautiful moments that uplifted me, though I must have cried a thousand tears. I sat for hours staring into the distance, clamped inside with a tightness in my chest and an ache that would not go away. I could not bear to see other women's babies. Everyday conversations seemed trite and I had no energy for them. I was consumed with the idea of suffering and my search for hope. I wrote down the words that came spitting out of my mouth when the longing filled me up. I bandaged my breasts so the milk would dry up quickly, and the milk came out in tears instead. I tried to share my pain with my partner. We were good together as we carried that heavy burden, but we also needed to process the loss in our own ways. Inevitably, there were times when we could not offer each other the support we needed.

I can't say when exactly, but the blistering pain gave way to something soft and melancholy, like a golden light at the end of the day or the feeling you have when you are alone on a bus, staring out the window at the scenery passing by. I still felt sad knowing we would never see Jacob grow up. I would never know if he had blue eyes like his sister or dark brown like his brother or if he was a swimmer, a surfer, a water polo player, or just liked to frolic in the water. It seemed unfair that he was missing out on all the ordinariness, the mystery, the rapture, and the turmoil of a life lived. But the bitterness was quelled inside me. It was replaced by a sweet sensation. Whenever I thought about him, I felt him alight, always in the same place, a warm and fleeting sensation on the tender spot just below my left shoulder. Then my thoughts would wander and he'd leave without a trace. I would lie quietly, looking up through the skylight, feeling the memory of him flit across the windowpane, and slowly I began to find peace.

In 1999, it was generally believed that naming a stillborn baby and keeping his memory alive was a healthy and potentially healing response. The days when women were encouraged not to see or hold their dead babies, when they were urged to move on and forget what had happened were gone. I don't know how those women kept their secrets for so long. I imagine a great wave of sorrow swelling in their breasts, held back against their better instincts. I met one of these mothers once. She was an old woman, probably in her late 80s judging by the wrinkles on her cheeks and the curve of her back. I was on my knees, hunched over with my back to her, digging in the soil where we had planted a memorial tree. She approached me and asked what I was doing. When I told her I planted flowers every Mother's Day to honour the memory of my baby, tears rolled down her face. She held my gaze for a moment before she told me that she, too, had given birth to a stillborn baby, 1 of 10 children she had birthed. She said it was the first time she had spoken about it since the night he died.

We never thought to bury our story. Including Jacob in our family narrative came naturally to all of us, even his little sister who blessed us with her welcomed arrival exactly one year minus three days after his birth.

Speaking his name and seeing it spelled out brought relief. At the cottage on Georgian Bay where we spent our happiest family times together, we named our boat *Jacob's Ladder*. We painted his name on a smooth rock perched at the highest point on the island. I would sit there on the craggy edge looking down over the great expanse of crystal water, whispering his name. In the city, the memorial tree and a park bench with a plaque bearing his name became a place of refuge for me and my husband when we were seeking solace from the world. We often celebrated his birthday by gathering at that spot. We hung a small red stocking for Jacob on the mantle at Christmastime and a white dove ornament with his name on the Christmas tree. Each one of us devised a private way of remembering him that helped transform the hurt into something poignant and meaningful.

When Jacob was born still, I was afraid that in losing him he would be lost to me. I befriended my grief when I needed to be with him night and day. When I realized his story did not end the day he was born, I found my way again. I discovered his sweet presence close by me, as a memory and a mystery I couldn't quite divine. I didn't feel any stronger, but I felt a breathless wonder at the remarkable journey of the monarch.

9

THE FIVE-YEAR PLAN

Sonal Champsee

THE PLAN

1. Get married
2. Buy house
3. Start and finish master's degree
4. Have two kids

YOUR WEDDING WAS small and beautiful. Even your parents admit you planned a lovely event, although you still have to stop your mother from doing her usual postmortem of how she could have planned things better. Your mother-in-law, fresh from the end of chemotherapy, cooed over your best friend's five-week-old baby.

You and your husband live in your separate condos at first; you're 35 and he's 41, and you're both settled in your own spaces. But as soon you buy a house, a fixer-upper with 100-year-old painted bricks and 40-year-old avocado green appliances, you pack and move and sell your old place in between coursework for your degree.

Your father, who is also your business partner and a real estate broker, wants to know why you need such a big house. He really means "Why aren't you living closer to us?" but you explain that the house has five bedrooms: a room for you and your husband to sleep in, a room each for an office, and two rooms for kids.

Both your parents are surprised. "Aren't you too old to have kids?"

You explain that all your friends had kids in their mid to late 30s, but your parents only know Indian families, and good Indian kids get married in their 20s. Your father persists. "But won't the child be mentally deficient? Won't it take some kind of medical miracle for you to have a baby?"

THE THINGS YOU DIDN'T KNOW

The plan is to lower the basement floor to build an apartment and at least renovate the kitchen and bathrooms before having a baby. You want a year of marriage before having kids. You're a little afraid of how having a baby will derail your degree and your nascent writing career and irrevocably change your life. You know you don't have a lot of time, but you want to do this sensibly, in an orderly way. Responsibly.

You blow the entire renovation budget and more on the basement. The clay drainage pipes shatter in the dig, and in the flooded muddy mess you find drowned sewer rats. The heat goes out on the night of your first reading of your first published work of fiction, and the hot water tank is punctured when you have the reading of your first play. Your front and back yards become repositories for construction debris and mud.

Everything takes too long and you turn 36. You begin trying to conceive, and you get bogged down in the issue of timing. All the advice you find is about normal, 28-day cycles, but you've never had one of those. In the last few years, your cycle has gone from short and slightly irregular to anywhere from 16 to 45 days. You blame it on stress.

You're well-educated, but you're surprised to discover that you have no idea when you ovulate. In a normal cycle, the follicular phase, when an egg grows, lasts about two weeks, followed by ovulation and a luteal phase that lasts another two weeks. But if you have a 16-day cycle, do you ovulate on Day 2 or Day 14? How long does it take to grow an egg in a follicle? When is a lining thick enough? You've heard of estrogen and progesterone from birth control pills, but what exactly do they do?

You look into the movie trope of taking your temperature and discover that temperature rises after ovulation, not before; it doesn't tell you when to try, but confirms the time has passed. You start peeing on ovulation predictor kits that test for a surge in the luteinizing hormone, or LH, which triggers ovulation. You've never heard of LH before.

Your family doctor finds out you're trying and orders a test for follicle-stimulating hormone, or FSH, on Day 3 of your cycle. You've never heard of FSH before either. Your results come back slightly but not concerningly high. Still, she refers you to a fertility clinic. "It can take a few months to get an appointment," she says. "So you may as well try to book one now."

The first appointment date is the day of the opening of your first play in Seattle. You move the appointment to two weeks later and already feel like a bad mother for choosing career over children.

The house is still full of boxes; you combined two households and your husband is a packrat. You refuse to unpack anything inessential, since you'll only have to pack it and move it when you renovate that part of the house. You keep the vases and the crystal and most of your books in boxes. Your husband drags his feet on decluttering. "Why don't we move this stuff to the second bedroom?" he says. "We aren't using it."

You refuse several times before you snap at him. "That's the baby's room. I don't want us to fill it up and get used to using it for stuff and then have to empty it all out when I get pregnant." The arguments stop. You move an old sofa in there, which the cats sleep on, but otherwise leave the room empty and waiting.

You still think having children is a choice you can make. Of course you do. They call it "birth control," as if you will magically get pregnant the moment you stop actively preventing it. You will learn this is not the case.

Before you see the fertility doctor, you draw the line at in vitro fertilization (IVF). "We aren't going to go crazy on this," you say to your husband. "We're just going to rule out anything simple and easy." You don't want to become one of those women who go crazy trying to have a baby, injecting themselves with hormones and blowing thousands of dollars. At this point, you fully expect the doctor to tell you it's just stress. You're under a lot of stress between work, school, the renovations, your parents, and sharing a household with another person for the first time in years.

The doctor is well dressed and pretty. She's Asian and you imagine that, like you, she is a child of immigrants. She speaks frankly and asks many questions and then orders several tests. For your husband, blood work and sperm tests. For you, blood work, transvaginal ultrasounds, and a sonohysterogram, which involves filling your uterus with saline and then checking for abnormalities. The numbers reveal you have diminished ovarian reserve. Your FSH is a touch high, your AMH — that's anti-Müllerian hormone — is normal, but your follicle count is very low. In plain English, your reproductive system looks more like that of a 42-year-old woman than a 37-year-old one. You are pissed off to realize that your parents were right about your being too old even though you are not actually too old.

There is reason to hope. You still ovulate regularly, and in fertility terms 37 isn't old, although egg quality typically declines rapidly after that point. You ask if there are any tests for quality but there are not. Medical science can only use age as a best guess.

The doctor prescribes Clomid and a few rounds of IUI — intrauterine insemination — and you're relieved by her cautious approach; you felt certain you were going to be pressured into expensive and unnecessary IVF treatments. The internet tells you that if IUI works, it usually works within three rounds. You are told to hope that Clomid will stimulate your ovaries into producing two or three follicles. An egg grows inside a follicle, and more eggs means better odds.

The internet tells you that some women get as many as six or seven follicles and have to cancel their cycle. You and your husband discuss selective reproduction. You take the warning about ovarian hyperstimulation syndrome — a potential and occasionally fatal side effect of stimulation — very seriously. You still think medical science has solutions. No one tells you that with your numbers, these possibilities are laughable.

Your in-laws, bless them, do not say one word to you about grandchildren, even though your husband is their only child. Your mother-in-law only repeats, "The children must make their own decisions." No one else is this polite.

At your in-laws' dinner table one night, your father interrupts a conversation about movies to say, "You know, in India, they have a really great system for surrogacy."

Your in-laws are confused, and your husband gives you an odd look. The two of you have never formally discussed keeping infertility treatments secret, but you haven't told anyone either. But you are used to your father's inability to read a room.

He continues: "It's so efficient. The citizenship is worked out before the baby is even born. Uncle Dinesh's son, Rohit — he and his wife had some problems. That's what they did. It's a very good system."

This is actually the fourth time your father has told you this, and you shut it down. "Yes, it sounds like a good system. If someone wants to do that."

Progress on the basement chugs along slowly. A concrete floor has been poured and the walls have been framed in, but when the plumbers replace the leaking cast iron stack, they discover there is no support under your toilet, and so you are left with a shower upstairs and a cramped powder room on the main floor. The electricians rewire the house, ripping into every wall and ceiling, revealing that your ductwork is covered in asbestos paper. On the advice of the removal company, you save $1,200 and rip it out yourselves, cutting wide gashes in the lathe and plaster walls. The baby's room — in fact, every room — has broken walls.

Every fertility treatment starts with a baseline monitoring appointment, blood tests, and a transvaginal ultrasound. The internet infertility groups you find call the ultrasound "being twatwanded" or "visiting the dildo-cam." You arrive at 7:00 a.m. to see the assembly line in full swing, but you don't yet know your place in it. You wait to get blood drawn, then strip from the waist down, put on a gown, and walk down the hall, back of your gown gaping, to wait for your ultrasound. The nurse, reading names off a clipboard, tells you that next time you should put on two gowns, one opening to the front, one to the back. You go into a dim room and put your feet in stirrups. A young doctor — not your doctor — rolls a condom over the wand, loads it up with gel, and inserts it. She moves it around, pressing on the inside of your hip to get a better view, and calls out numbers to the nurse. Then you're hustled out of there without knowing what any of those numbers mean. You wait for a nurse, who hands you a prescription for Clomid and tells you to start taking it tonight. You ask questions, but she can't answer them because she's not your doctor, but you aren't going to see your doctor. *Is this normal?*

Other women on the internet complain about their Clomid symptoms, but you feel nothing, and when you go for monitoring a few days later, there's only one follicle, the same as what you could do on your own. Before leaving the ultrasound room you ask the doctor when the IUI will be. She says usually not for another week. You explain you usually ovulate very early, but she tells you Clomid changes that. A nurse calls that night and tells you your blood work shows a surge in LH. You're ovulating and need to go for IUI tomorrow.

IUI is in a different room, brightly lit, and the stirrups are covered with bright red oven mitts for padding and warmth. The internet tells you to carry on as normal, but, conflictingly, to take it easy and keep your feet up. You wear warm socks just in case they will bring warm blood back to your uterus and help with implantation, and you eat pineapple core — not the flesh, only the core — for exactly five days afterward. None of this has any science behind it, but you try it even though it seems ridiculous.

None of it works.

For your second IUI, they try the highest dose of Clomid. Your second monitoring appointment is the day before Christmas, and the clinic is closed on Christmas. You ask the doctor — a different one again — when your IUI might be and he says not for a week, chuckling like it's a silly question. You try to explain that this happened last time; he should look at your chart and see, but you're ushered out of the room so the next woman can come in. Still, your doctor has left a note to give you a trigger shot — an injection of hCG hormone that mimics the LH surge — in case the last time was a weird fluke. You are shown how to use it and will be told when to take it.

But like last time, the nurse calls to say your LH surged on its own and you are ovulating, but to take the trigger shot anyway. You are instructed to have intercourse at home.

You've never injected yourself and at first you want your husband to do it, but you take over because you're afraid his nerves will make you more nervous. You line up the sharp steel point at 90 degrees to a pinch of belly skin. The hardest part is getting over the idea that you are supposed to avoid sticking sharp objects into yourself.

You're still not pregnant, but your period doesn't come when expected. After more monitoring, more blood tests, and more dates with the dildo-cam, they tell you to wait it out, which means more waiting before you can try again. Your period is three weeks late, but no one tells you what happened or why.

You go through your calendar, your posts in infertility groups, and your memory and start writing down every piece of data. You make an Excel spreadsheet and look for patterns. It's clear no one else is keeping track for you.

After baseline monitoring for the third IUI, you come home and work on writing assignments on the old couch in the future nursery; the third-floor room you were using as your office is uninsulated and too cold. The phone rings and the nurse tells you not to take Clomid. "Your FSH is fifty-eight."

"What does that mean? What's wrong?"

She can't answer your questions because only the doctor can do that. The IUI is cancelled but you can try at home with an ovulation predictor kit. You call to make an appointment with your doctor. The medical secretary tells you that you're lucky; there's a cancellation and she can see you in a week. You later find out that there's always a cancellation when it's bad news.

They say never consult Dr. Google, but you do, and everything you find about Day 3 FSH of 58 says something about menopause. You are only 37. Your FSH at your first appointment was 9.8. You've been led to believe that your problems are mild. What is going on now?

At the appointment, you discover your Google-diagnostic skills are pretty good. You are not, technically, in menopause, but your menopause-like levels of FSH indicate that there is no point in giving you any fertility medications. All stimulation medications increase FSH to make more follicles, but your FSH is already so high, medication won't make a difference. You ask, "How come it was lower before? Why did it spike?"

"It varies from cycle to cycle, but your highest number tends to be predictive of how things will go." The doctor never answers the question of why, because the whys are unknown.

"What about IVF?" you ask, even though Google has already answered this question.

The doctor shakes her head. "I'd estimate your chances with IVF to be between five percent and ten percent."

IVF success is highly correlated with the number of follicles they can stimulate the body into producing. More follicles, more eggs, more chances. Most of the medication used pumps the body full of FSH to try to get 10 or 12 eggs, but you'd be lucky to get 2. Very few eggs become babies. This isn't because of IVF, but is mostly because of what happens naturally. Only 80 percent of eggs fertilize. Then only 50 percent of those survive to become five-day blastocysts, which is when they are frozen or transferred back into the uterus. Only 30 percent of them will implant. You wonder how it is that any of them manage to live.

Your doctor asks if you've considered donor eggs. You didn't cry when Google suggested this, but now your eyes fill up with tears. Google also told you that South Asian donors are rare in North America. You find a news article from a clinic out west explaining that in those cases, they try to find a Hispanic or Indigenous American donor, as those turn out close enough. Close enough doesn't seem like enough.

MANAGING ENTROPY

Your mother-in-law's cancer comes back after four years. The five-year survival rate of her cancer is very low, but you still somehow imagined her playing with your children. She begins chemotherapy again, and your husband sits on her hospital bed and tells her about the fertility treatments. She's the first to know, and she's happy, because after that awkward dinner with your father, she thought you didn't want children at all. She was so sad about this but never said a word.

The thing with 5 percent odds is that they aren't zero, but it would cost you thousands of dollars to bet on those odds. What's the price tag for a child? There is no test for egg quality, but if IVF fails more than statistically expected, you can conclude it was probably due to egg quality. How do you put a price tag on failure? You become obsessed with your own data. Statistics was your worst subject in math, but you get your husband to teach you how to calculate cumulative odds and you run the numbers over and over again.

The question of trying is no longer about having a baby. You are probably not going to have a baby. Instead, it is about not having regrets. You need to be able to look back and see that you tried everything. You run the numbers and work out how many times you're willing to try before you can walk away in peace.

You seek out a second opinion from a doctor at the most cutting-edge clinic you can find, although given that you are older than the first baby born via IVF, the cutting edge is a rapidly moving target. You don't bring your medical records — you don't want your original doctor to know — but run through your spreadsheet and astonish the new doctor with the details you remember. The new doctor concurs with your original doctor, but agrees that it makes no sense to move on to donor eggs without trying your own. "Miracles happen."

You like him because he listens and explains things, drawing diagrams on paper and openly admitting what is unknown or untested. He wishes you luck and gives you his card, saying to email him and let him know how it goes. You believe he sincerely wants to know.

You go back to your original doctor, saying you want to try IVF. She demurs, repeating odds and asking about donor scenarios. But eventually she agrees to try.

You tell everyone that you're starting IVF and your odds are terrible so it probably won't work. You put it on Facebook. Twenty people reach out to you to say that they, too, sought fertility treatments. You had no idea. You start fertility acupuncture, and two friends from university tell you not to buy into the snake oil; you should trust medical science instead. You explain that medical science can't help you, but they still treat you like you're planning to inject your eyeballs with heroin. You tell them they can be supportive or they can fuck off. Neither of them are your friends anymore.

Your cousin tells you that she had multiple miscarriages and took Clomid to conceive, and then explains that she couldn't possibly be your surrogate because it would be too weird. You are simultaneously annoyed and furious. You don't need a surrogate, and a history of miscarriages would make her a bad candidate anyway, but how dare she preemptively refuse? What if you had needed one?

Your mother-in-law reveals that she tried for seven years, but a doctor gave her "some hormones" and she got pregnant with her son, your husband. You figure out that it must have been Clomid.

Your mother suggests adoption from India. "I could pick one up the next time I go." You explain that adoption is much more complicated than that, but she doesn't take it in. "You don't want to get pregnant. It's too much trouble. This way is much easier." You explain again that it isn't, and tell her about egg donation. You want her to be prepared if you go that route. She decides that your cousin's wife, who is nothing like you, would be perfect. "I'll tell her next time I'm in India."

At your first baseline monitoring appointment, the nurse has trouble getting a vein and eventually does the draw from your wrist. She asks if you're excited.

You're not but you try to joke it off. "I don't think anyone is excited to stab themselves with needles."

She admonishes you. "It's very exciting. Think about the baby!"

You want to scream at her and ask her if she understands what the numbers on your chart mean. You don't understand how a person can work at a fertility clinic and still think IVF always leads to a baby. But you say nothing. She draws your blood. You get twatwanded and go home.

After the appointment, you get a phone call telling you not to inject yourself with the expensive hormones. "You have an estrogen-producing cyst on the right."

You ask questions, but they have no answers. They only tell you that you cannot do IVF because the cyst will interfere with the medication, but you can try again next month.

The next month, you have an estrogen-producing cyst on the left. Cancelled again.

The next month, you have an estrogen-producing cyst on the right, but the doctor doing the ultrasound is your doctor. "Come back in two days, and we'll see if it resolves."

Two days later, the cyst is gone. You never thought you'd be happy to stab yourself daily with needles. You go back for monitoring two days later and then head up to the cottage. The clinic calls. "Stop taking medications," says the nurse. "You've already ovulated."

You try asking questions but they have no answers and cell reception is poor. You make an appointment to see your doctor. Luckily, there's a cancellation. The pants-on appointments are always bad news.

Your doctor explains: "What we thought were cysts are actually follicles that developed too early, out of sync with the rest of your cycle."

Eggs. Potential babies. Three chances, lost. You are angry to the point of tears that they can be so cavalier about skipping months, as if you have eggs in abundance and all the time in the world. You ask about different protocols, about the possibility of suppression medications to prevent the follicles from developing early. Your doctor shakes her head. "Now that you've tried three IVF cycles, have you thought about donor eggs?"

You don't consider three cancelled cycles trying IVF at all, and you walk out of the clinic crying. You fumble in your purse for the business card of the other doctor. You call and get an appointment in two days, and then call the clinic you just left and ask them to send over your medical records. Having settled on a new plan, you're calm again.

The new doctor explains. Follicles and cysts look the same on an ultrasound. Follicles produce estrogen but so do some cysts. The follicle they saw must have ovulated, then disappeared, and then became a corpus luteum, which produces progesterone, confirming ovulation. All of these look the same on an ultrasound. The clarity is a relief. They were not withholding answers. They were guessing.

Your writing desk now sits in the future nursery. Writing on the couch hurts your back. The contractors are working in the basement in fits and starts; you can't stay on top of ordering material for them. You should be working on your thesis but you can't focus. The house, with its mud and gravel yard and the inside full of dust and broken plaster and cat-fur tumbleweeds, looks like depression.

The acupuncturist you see specializes in fertility. It's a relief to talk to him about IVF without having to explain the medical details; you've all but completely given up on talking to anyone else. He kicks your ass about your thesis and holds you accountable for writing deadlines. You have no idea if acupuncture is helping, but you look forward to the weekly chat.

There are no gowns at the new clinic. You strip from the waist down in the ultrasound room and wrap a paper sheet around yourself. Afterward, you see a doctor — as usual not necessarily your doctor — instead of a nurse. Otherwise, the routine is the same.

One day you leave the clinic only to find out your contractor asked for the wrong-sized door. You hop on the subway, borrow your mother's van, pick up the door, and go to exchange it. It's time to inject, so you sit in the steamy van in the parking lot of Home Depot, mix diluent into powdered Menopur, and inject yourself. You feel badass. You half expect someone to call and report a junkie shooting up drugs.

You decide to have a party for your 38th birthday, to celebrate your broken house, and to force yourself to clean. You unpack the boxes of crystal you've kept packed for three years while waiting for the end of the renovations. You no longer know when you'll be done.

The cycle runs long. Despite the injections, nothing is growing. Your doctor advises you to wait it out, and eventually one follicle grows. There is no miracle that makes you grow more. You're given a trigger shot to take precisely 36 hours before your egg retrieval. You and your husband go to the clinic, you're given an IV for twilight sleep, and your husband dons a surgical cap and gown and goes in with you.

Afterward, you hazily remember something went wrong. They wheeled you out of the room without retrieving anything. Your doctor explains: even though you took medications to suppress ovulation, you ovulated through it. The one precious egg is lost somewhere in your Fallopian tubes.

That night, your husband is called to the hospital. Your mother-in-law's chemotherapy has not been going well. There are lumps growing in her throat and blocking her airway. After much hasty discussion in the emergency room, she gets a tracheotomy. She cannot speak with the tube in. No one tells her that she'll have this tube for months.

Every problem in your life you have solved by declaring war on it, but you are in a war with no allies. Your friends sympathize but lack the medical knowledge to keep them from asking stupid questions or suggesting that you just relax. Your husband is now overwhelmed by his mother's illness. Your parents are worse than useless. You have your doctor, your acupuncturist, and the internet.

Your life now consists of bouncing back and forth between the clinic and the hospital. You keep writing cheques to contractors, but you're still in a house with holes and no full bathrooms. Landscapers come to lay out new paths, but the weeds have taken over what's left of the mud piles. You and your husband agree to ignore the marriage, because neither of you have the energy. There are medical questions without answers everywhere you turn. Infertility seems so much less than cancer. You're not dying. But you can't make life happen.

At your next baseline, the doctor — not your doctor, another one — tells you that you have a cyst and to keep taking estrogen to see if it resolves, but you might need to cancel the cycle.

You explain that this happened at your last clinic, that they weren't cysts but early follicles, that your cycle goes out of sync. He tells you it's a cyst and that you should take estrogen. You tell him to look at your chart, look at your clinic records, because what if this one is an egg? He tells you it's a cyst and that you should take estrogen. You're talking to a wall.

You're angry but you leave the clinic with a prescription for estrogen. You sit outside the doors on a sunny bench near a coffee shop patio. You start writing an email to your doctor, but midway through, he walks up from down the street. You tell him that you were about to send him a message, and he says he's seen the results and sits on the bench beside you to talk.

He listens as you explain. "I'm afraid we might miss a chance. That this is actually an egg."

He understands, although he still believes it's a cyst. But he tells you cyst aspiration and egg retrieval are the same procedure and suggests trying it. "If nothing else, for your peace of mind." He sends you home with a trigger shot, and the aspiration/retrieval is scheduled for two days later, on the fifth day of your cycle. Far too early for an egg in a normal cycle, but nothing about you is normal.

A different doctor performs this and an embryologist is standing by in case. You are in twilight sleep, but you hear someone say there's an egg.

Your doctor is surprised and says you were right. You tell him to cheer up — maybe he'll get a case study out of this. The egg fertilizes, proving that it is viable, and grows to two cells before arresting. The embryologist thought it might be slightly immature. You look at the photo; you created a life, even if it didn't last.

The next cycle goes long, like your first one. Your mother-in-law gets sicker, trying different chemotherapies, until eventually they stop trying and start talking about palliative care. But she does not want to stop trying, even though there is nothing left to try. She tells you, writing on a pad of paper, that she dreamed you were pregnant. "I was so happy, I felt like I was in ninth heaven." She rushes you out of there so you won't be late for acupuncture, and afterward you work on your thesis because the deadline is close.

The next day she dies.

It is a Friday.

Death comes with a lot of paperwork, and you take that on so that your husband and father-in-law can grieve. You email your thesis adviser and tell her you have to delay your first draft. The following Monday, you go in for monitoring. Your one follicle is nearly mature, and you calculate that the retrieval will probably be on the day of the funeral. Medication could delay ovulation, but you're on a special, low-cost, no-medication plan. Your doctor is away for Rosh Hashanah, but the doctor you speak to remembers your bizarrely early egg retrieval. Still, he suggests skipping this cycle and waiting for a better one.

You tell him you don't have better cycles and about your late mother-in-law's dream. You are not skipping anything if there's a chance. He tells you to talk to your own doctor and leaves the room without giving his condolences.

You email your doctor and see him the next day, and he pulls some strings to let you take the medication. The retrieval is the day after the funeral. The egg doesn't fertilize.

On the day of the funeral, landscapers visit your house to lay a fresh green lawn. At least your house looks beautiful on the outside.

You go through three more cycles. The first is another bizarrely early cycle that has your doctor apologizing to the nurses for nonstandard requests. But it results in a perfect eight-cell embryo for the freezer.

The second, you ovulate before your baseline appointment. The third is unusually normal, and results in a six-cell embryo for transfer.

Your doctor recommends transferring the frozen eight-cell embryo along with the fresh one, but you are afraid. That embryo is safe in the freezer, but once you transfer, that might be it. Eight-cells might be the closest you ever come to being a parent. There won't be school photos or wedding photos, but at least you have a photo of eight perfect cells.

You transfer both.

One becomes your son.

Every child is supposedly a miracle, but your child proved two doctors wrong by merely existing. On your last appointment, you thank your doctor. He shrugs and says, "I'm just the waiter." He can't get a case study out of this, since there is no way to prove if this came from the normal cycle or the bizarrely early one he'd done on your request. But both of you know, deep down, which one it was.

THE AFTERMATH

You live in the least baby-safe house on earth and so you rush through everything, finishing the day before your due date. Having a bathroom again is a wonder. You put off the final draft of your thesis; you need a livable house more than you need this degree.

Your son is the most amazing thing you've ever seen, but there is no happily-ever-after ride into the sunset. You spent longer being infertile than you spend being pregnant; you can't wrap your head around the change. Your pregnancy is textbook and boring.

While you're pregnant, friends give you their old baby gear, and you shut it in the nursery because you cannot connect with the idea that you are actually having a baby. Everyone is excited and squealing, but you don't want to talk about it. They ask you what you most look forward to but your mind goes blank. Not from fear. Many of the women from your internet groups are terrified they will lose the baby, but you are stuck on the unreality. You are not afraid of losing the baby because you cannot even imagine the baby. The only thing you want is for him to really exist. The first thought you have when he emerges from your body is, *How did this baby get here?*

You were prepared for the hard work of parenting, but you have an easy child, and you are surprised that it's also fun. After the first hectic months, you plug away at your thesis again and eventually graduate. Your parents say nothing. Your father-in-law is proud. You don't fly out to your graduation ceremony because the idea of travelling with a baby feels like too much.

Everyone comments on his beautiful grey eyes. You assume the colour will change to brown, since your side is all brown eyes and isn't brown dominant? But they never change. You wonder about a mix-up at the clinic; perhaps it was not your egg after all. You realize that wouldn't change anything about how you feel about him, but you still consult Google and are relieved to discover the genetic basis of eye colour is considerably more complicated than you thought.

People start asking you when you're going to have a second child, and you want to slap them for not understanding that you gave birth to a miracle. There is no formula for repeating miracles. You will always be infertile.

Still, as your son outgrows his baby clothes, you can't bear to give them away. Your maternity clothes are still in a box in your room. What if you have another? You know this is almost certainly impossible, but in your head, the plan was always two kids. Your writing desk sits in the empty room. The odds were against you before and you are now 40 years old, so the odds will be worse. You could calculate them. Lightning doesn't strike twice. Does it?

10

MOVING OUT OF INFERTILITY

Sarah Coulson

INFERTILITY SHRINKS YOUR WORLD. It steals your life. It traps you in a desperate, hard, miserable place where the only thing that matters is whether your period comes, what the outcome of your next appointment is, whether you're finally going to succeed and get the pregnancy and the baby you so desperately want.

Infertility is a risky investment fund that takes your carefully hoarded hope, time, and money and drains it on the promise that one day you, too, will be the proud parent of one of the adorable pudgy babies pictured on fertility clinic walls.

Infertility is a place you live — a glass-domed city, full of hopeful, desperate neighbours. You don't really pack your things and move there. You just find yourself there, a bit at a time. Once you're there, though, the knowledge of your new address permeates your mind. You can look out of Infertility, and some people seem to leave, but you're never really sure if you're going to be one of them. From inside, you can see only one way out, and the key is shaped like a positive pregnancy test.

You never intended to live in Infertility. You pack your life up for parenthood, intending to journey in a timely manner through the world of pregnancy: nausea, maybe; fecundity; looser joints; swollen ankles; doulas; midwives; birth plans; and watching out for predictable roadblocks like gestational diabetes. You figure this will, in due time, let you move to a place called Parenthood, where late-night feedings, worrying about sniffles, teething, baby's first everything, little gummy baby smiles, perfect tiny feet, and that new baby smell are fixtures of the landscape. All you have to do is get there.

Somewhere along the way, you take a detour and wind up in Infertility. It is not a neighbourhood with a great deal to recommend. You never know how long you're going to stay.

Of course, I didn't intend to move to Infertility. I was going to be a parent. I was always going to be a parent. I had a plan: find a job with benefits; find a donor — someone who seemed genetically plausible, who I could trust enough to share bodily fluids with, and who didn't have any interest in co-parenting; have unprotected sex; get pregnant; and become a mother. It was a good plan, sort of. I talked about it with my grandmother, and she said, "Make sure you have a good lawyer for that donor man, so you don't wind up parenting with someone useless." (I did find a good lawyer. I drew up an agreement, and promised the world would never know who my donor was. He promised me he didn't want to be a father.)

I told my mother and she said, "You know I'll support you, Sarah, but doesn't that seem like it's going to be hard?"

I figured it would be easier than finding someone I wanted to parent with forever.

I found the job with the benefits. First step achieved.

It was now or never, and *never* sounded like failure, so my donor and I got our blood tests and started having unprotected sex.

I got my period.

I tried again.

I got my period.

If you've moved to Infertility, you know what the road in looks like. My journey wasn't very different. I started charting my temperature and cervical mucus. I did not realize it at the time, but this was my introduction to the bizarre snow-globe neighbourhood of Infertility. I would spend the next several years moving deeper and deeper into it, never getting any closer to the exit.

Sex became a matter of timing rather than desire, a project rather than a recreation. Each month, I greeted my period with weary frustration.

The next stage in my relocation to Infertility occurred in my doctor's office. She agreed with me that there was no obvious reason for me not to be pregnant yet. We booked some tests. And just like that, instead of living in Pregnancy and Parenthood, I had moved to Infertility.

The neighbours were kind and generous with their advice: don't get too stressed out, eat pineapple, try in the morning, try before bed, hug your knees to your chest after he's done. Have orgasms.

Infertility is a small neighbourhood, filled with people doing the same things: Attending doctor's appointments. Getting blood taken. Having more purposeful, hopeful intercourse (with desperate orgasms). Doggedly tracking basal body temperatures and cervical mucus. Counting days.

From my new residence inside the snow-globe landscape of tracking, testing, consulting, trying, waiting, and dealing with monthly disappointment, I could look out and see other people whose lives did not appear to be dominated by my struggle to get pregnant. Other people did not appear to be struggling to get pregnant at all. Co-workers, friends, and cousins announced their pregnancies and went about gestating, nesting, and delivering babies with seeming abandon.

Outside the snow-globe neighbourhood, things completely unrelated to my, or anyone else's, fertility continued to happen: people moved house, had parties, lived their lives.

Eventually, residents of Infertility seem to wind up at the fertility clinic. Its walls are adorned with photos of your destination — photos of happy families, tired and complete with their squiggly babies.

Fertility clinics never show pictures of the people who didn't succeed. So when you visit one, you imagine yourself only as one of the successes. You feel like you're in the immigration office for Parenthood, and all you have to do is fill out the forms, take the tests, jump through the hoops, and demonstrate that you, too, are fit to move to Parenthood. Of course, there are no photos of the people who never got their visas.

Nobody wants a reminder of the failures. Nobody wants to hear the stories of the hopeful would-be parents who poured themselves into their dreams of a family, who did everything they could, and, after years of trying, years of medical intervention, years dedicated to a project, just … didn't succeed. Nobody wants a picture of giving up.

I was a good applicant. I did the things. I took the tests. I kept trying and trying and trying. Until, one day, I just didn't.

Infertility has one apparent exit. Another word for this kind of place might be *trap*. Some people get out of the trap. Some people get stuck. While you're there, getting to that exit consumes you. All your best efforts can keep you trapped in Infertility for years. While you're there, the rest of the world goes to new destinations. People may express sympathy, but no one stops and waits until you've found your way to Parenthood. Your friends — the ones with whom you were going to raise children — have kids, and their kids get older. Your employment may change. My good, steady job with benefits up and disappeared. My donor got tired and severed ties. My second donor's life became unexpectedly busy, making scheduling an issue.

I met someone. Dating turned into a relationship. He had a kid and didn't want another one. Many fraught conversations left us at an impasse: I kept doing what I had been doing, he kept wishing I wouldn't, and we stopped talking about it. Something was going to have to give.

Something gave.

On a Tuesday afternoon, I had an appointment to go over some test results and maybe get some answers. I gathered my papers, put on my shoes, but didn't go.

The pictures of babies on the clinic wall danced in my imagination, and in that moment none of them looked like they might be mine. The clinic did not seem to offer a way out of Infertility for me: it merely offered more of the same. Where were the people who had found a different way out? How many had given up? Well, one that I knew of. Not enough people talk about the other road out.

When momentous decisions happen, sometimes they don't happen all at once. I didn't go to an appointment. I'll never know why I'm infertile. A little bit at a time, I made my life about something other than trying to conceive. I stopped eating pineapple and I will never eat it again. I stopped tracking my temperature and cervical mucus. All that information about my cycle didn't do me a lick of good anyway, and now I could drink the coffee that my beloved brought first thing in the morning without fear or anger. I didn't call my donor when my supposedly fertile period began. I bought him a card and had him over for dinner sometime around Day 16 a couple of months later, to say thank you. Sex with a loving partner became something we did for fun, because the mood took us.

While you're trapped in Infertility, life sometimes presents you with routes to parenthood you hadn't planned on. When I'd been stuck in cycles and cycles of trying, I had also been holding myself back from committing fully to the family I had already gained: the one with the truly decent guy and the kid he and his ex-wife were raising. While I was holding on to dreams of a baby of my own, this other family was right outside the borders I'd set up for all of us.

It turns out that you can walk out of Infertility at any time. The place is full of crossroads, and a lot of those alternate routes will take you elsewhere. You may never find the road to Pregnancy. Sometimes, though, life gives you alternate routes to Parenthood. Maybe they don't look like the one you had mapped out. Maybe Parenthood isn't really the neighbourhood you thought it was going to be, with first birthdays, first teeth, and first steps. Sometimes you leap over those milestones and build your own further along.

I wound up doing all the sorts of activities that parents do: going to teacher meetings, writing letters to principals, putting on birthday parties at bowling alleys and circus schools, rolling fondant for extravagant birthday cakes, sewing costumes late into the night, helping with homework, attending school plays and beginner recorder recitals (for my sins), going on family vacations, enduring tantrums, practising positive discipline, and doing school pick-ups. I'm That Parent: the one who noisily reminds schools and community groups and other parents that there are all kinds of valid ways to make a family and that not every parent is a mom or a dad.

I make it sound so easy, now, don't I? I skipped an appointment and made a decision, and the family I had been ignoring was just waiting for me. That would be a nice, tidy story. It would also be only half true.

The other half of the truth is that moving out of Infertility was hard. The missed appointment was the beginning of a process. To stop trying was pretty easy. To stop wishing was not. When I left Infertility, I carried with me years' worth of bitterness, frustration, resentment, and plain old sadness. I still get quietly angry when people I don't like announce their pregnancies. I definitely still want to hold and cuddle all the babies I can (except for the babies of people I don't like, because that would be weird). For a long time, I greeted my period each month with weary resentment, not for the pain and mess and general nuisance, but because a tiny, irrational part of me held out bizarre hope for some kind of weird fertility miracle. I still haven't gone on hormonal birth control, even if it might help my cramps. For a long time, it was because doing so would feel like completely, utterly shutting the door to any kind of impossible miracle. Now it's just because I've been off birth control for so long I can't imagine going back on it.

Getting over *myself* was not a smooth or easy process. With so many years invested in a baby who was now never going to be conceived, I had to figure out how to be okay with something that felt a lot like failure. I had failed. I didn't try hard enough. I didn't start early enough. I didn't find the right donors.

Learning to not resent people who had managed to become pregnant or, worse yet, people who became pregnant *without even trying* took some doing. Back in the early days in Infertility, when friends had apologized for getting pregnant without really even trying, I had blithely said, "Oh, don't be silly. It's not like there's only a finite number of babies in the baby pot and your baby means there are fewer left to go around."

Blithe, not-yet-trapped me was right, but bitter, tired me still railed at the unfairness of it all: I had tried so hard for so long, and I would have been such a good parent to a baby. I had done all this reading; I had worked so hard; it was so unfair.

Even now, years on, I still mourn the baby I'll never get to raise. It was only very recently that I met news of an acquaintance's long-hoped-for pregnancy with a genuine cry of gladness for her, completely absent of any twinge of resentment or wistfulness. On a scale of 1 to 10, where 1 is "still devastated and stuck" and 10 is "perfectly happy with the choices I made," I would have to say I'm at about an 8. Eight times out of 10, I like the parenting neighbourhood I wound up in. That's almost 20 hours out of every 24. How many people can say they're that close to okay with any choice they've made?

Moving out of Infertility turned out to be a messy, lengthy, and complicated process. It meant letting go of a lot: eating pineapple (no regrets), tracking my basal body temperature (also no regrets), a friend's baby furniture kept in her basement for me (small regret), a small part of my heart and a long-held vision of how my life was going to be (significant regret that shrank over time). It also meant embracing a whole other set of choices and outcomes: stepparenting and juggling the demands of four parents and eight pairs of grandparents. My family is tied to one city because my kid's other family is here. Decisions about school, vacations, summer camps, after-school programs, orthodontia, and anything else monumental is split four ways. I wanted to be a solo parent because I didn't trust anyone else to do things right; now I have to trust three other people, only one of whom I chose. (That they also have to trust me is not lost on me.)

My kid will never look even a little bit like me, so I have to find my influence in his behaviour: his choices of words; his belief that people need to take care of each other; his ability to notice when a book or movie lacks representation of people other than white men; and also his ability to fritter away time and get lost in nonessential tasks, argue for the sake of arguing, and not get out of bed early enough to get anywhere on time. There's a little bit of me in all of those, even if nobody will ever see me in his physique. Embracing the family that life brought me has meant smiling when people comment on the lack of physical resemblance between us or can't tell which kid is mine or where I belong at parent-child events. It's meant pulling up a third chair at parent-teacher interviews and fighting with schools to get my name put on email distribution lists.

With all that, I don't really have time to waste being sad about the other path out of Infertility. Moving out meant reclaiming my body, my life, and my future, all the while leaving a part of my heart behind. I think I finally realized I was over it all this past winter when I started the paperwork to donate a kidney to a friend. As long as I needed my body for a possible pregnancy, I could never have risked a live organ donation. But now that my body belongs to me alone, and not a hypothetical fetus, I can choose to take risks knowing that the family I have and love supports me.

Maybe I will never be 100 percent over it. I think I'm fine with that, too. My family's portrait graces my screensaver, my office walls, my kid's grandparents' walls, and our respective social media accounts. The clinic can keep its babies and the beginnings they represented for their families. We've found our own path.

11

MY SO-CALLED INFERTILE LIFE

Nicole Armstrong

IN 2010, AT THE AGE OF 28, I had a great career and I was soon to marry a great guy who also happened to be a handsome firefighter. We'd been lifelong friends and our relationship was effortless. We had both been fortunate in the way our parents had raised us; we were independent, motivated individuals who genuinely loved and respected each other's accomplishments. My parents had introduced me to the concept of excellence in achievement at an early age and expected it in everything my siblings and I did: school, sports, careers, social lives, love lives. Basically everything.

As a result of my DNA and upbringing, I am a compulsive perfectionist. Throughout my life, I have put a lot of pressure on myself to succeed, and when life throws me a curveball, I don't believe in waiting for the problem to figure itself out. I am compelled to take it on, fix it, and move on. Through my experiences with my so-called infertile life, I have learned many important lessons about the person I am and the person I want to be.

Because I am a perfectionist, not being able to solve for the missing variable of our unexplained infertility was, over time, a detriment to my life, my marriage, and my happily ever after. The constant thinking and problem-solving was mental and emotional agony. The fact that I couldn't magically solve the chromosomal XX/XY procreation equation the old-fashioned way, with a few extra-premium prenatal vitamins, took its toll.

Midway into 2011, we decided to start "not trying" to get pregnant. No luck putting one past the goalie the first few months. Without concern, we kept "not trying," believing that our youth and good exercise and eating habits would let it happen when it was meant to happen.

But as time went on, I started to feel the pressure and just wanted a medical professional to fix my damn infertility. I booked an appointment with my gynaecologist in the new year and resolved to enjoy the pre-baby time I had left. We scheduled a long weekend in New York City for a combination Christmas/30th birthday celebration. In February we flew out — it was time to forget the fertility frustrations.

A year of new beginnings, 2012. This would be the year of the Armstrong baby. Shortly into the new year, I was sitting in the exam room waiting for my gynaecologist, a middle-aged balding man who was minimally interested in solving the mystery of my infertility. Without much consideration of the issue, he recommended a fertility drug meant to increase the growth and release of mature follicles in each cycle. After my own research, I determined that this pharmaceutical sounded safe enough. I casually joked with my colleagues that maybe we would have twins, that with a two-for-one deal we could make up for lost time. The five months spent taking this supposed baby-creating medicine were filled with intense headaches, mood swings, acne, period tracking, temperature taking, and, most of all, being a constant party pooper. "No, sorry, just one drink tonight. I'm ovulating, and having fun will probably lessen my chances of getting pregnant."

By now, six months of "not trying" plus five months of failed pharmaceutically enhanced trying equalled what was most likely a problem. A problem amplified by the fact that all my newly wedded friends were getting pregnant on the first try. Subconsciously, my genetic code was taking the reins and steering me into my preconditioned problem-solving mode.

After about 13 months with no luck, I could hear my biological clock ticking. I sensed that we might need help in the baby-making department. I made an appointment for my husband, Chad, to see our family doctor. Our family doctor referred him to a male-specimen testing lab in the Greater Toronto Area and advised him, "Just keep trying. You are young and healthy. Try not to worry. Sometimes it takes a little longer."

Two or three weeks later, male factor infertility was confirmed. My husband's sperm motility was far below average. Then came the tears and self-pity that, of course, I had married "that guy." *Divorce?* No, too soon. Rather, I resolved that I would help my husband's sperm motility improve through a stricter diet and reduced caffeine and by keeping his testicles at the proper temperature. No more lazy swimmers for my uterus. I mentally prepared myself for my version of Male Infertility Problem-Solving 101.

One of the thousands of tidbits of advice for the infertile available via the World Wide Web includes seeing a naturopath. As the pharmaceutical drugs hadn't worked, it felt right to try the holistic way. Within a week, we had an appointment to see a local naturopath, before which we filled out a 35-page health questionnaire. Before we had even met, this holistic stranger knew a lot about us. At our first three-hour appointment, we spent approximately the equivalent of a monthly car payment learning how to attempt to fix our fertility problem the natural way. We committed to a cleanse to help clean our bodies of infertile impurities. We agreed to eliminate a lot of the deliciously toxic food and drink that we admitted to indulging in. We learned to replace gluten, dairy, caffeine, and sugar with whole-food eating.

While Chad had a harder time at first, he learned to appreciate the changes we were making together. I wouldn't say that I enjoyed the early days of radical changes in diet, exercise, caffeinating, and casual drinking, but one of us had to stay motivated to try to solve our infertility problems. At the first casual meals we shared with friends and family, we tried to explain why we were making these changes: "We're mildly concerned about our infertility and we're just trying out an altered diet to see if it boosts our chances at conception."

Of course, not everyone agreed with our reasons for changing our diet and lifestyle, but what did they know? The most common advice we heard from couples with no experience in infertility was "Just relax and it'll happen."

After six-ish months of our super-clean eating and living protocol, still no baby. The frustration between my husband and me was mounting. We had both tried to submit to the process of fertilizing our fertility, but nothing was working. The pressure we were putting on ourselves grew heavier, and we agreed to seek help from a reproductive medicine clinic.

In July 2012 we handed over our fertility problems to a reputable reproductive doctor. He was a straight-shooting, Converse shoe–wearing silver fox. Entering the clinic felt like walking into an exclusive private club, a secret from our friends and colleagues. As I looked around the waiting room, it was alarming to see how many couples were also having trouble conceiving a child.

At our first appointment with the newest member of the Baby Armstrong Problem-Solving Team, we were given the rundown on preliminary testing and how the results of blood work, ultrasounds, and microscopic observations of our genetic material would dictate our treatment protocol. I respected Dr. Silver Fox's confidence, and his no-nonsense philosophy was refreshing, especially considering that in the last year no provincially funded medical practitioner had been overly eager to solve our infertility equation.

The battery of tests confirmed that we were both fertilely imperfect. We already knew my husband had backward swimmers, but we now learned that my uterus had a septum.

Dr. Silver Fox explained the process needed to repair it, noting that it would give a fertilized egg a better chance of nestling in, without being cramped for space. This newly introduced solution would put having a baby on hold for half a year; it was my introduction to the incredibly slow-moving process of reproductive treatment. With a surgery date late in 2012, I resigned to enjoy my time not pregnant. What was a few more months?

Our friends and family knew that baby-making was on hold due to a repair under my hood. While explaining this step in our journey, I was happy to add that my mother had passed the faulty septum on to me, and therefore my part of the infertility was inherent — nothing I could have done about it.

With my septum repaired, the next phase in our fertility-fix program would be intrauterine insemination. Together we agreed to give Baby Armstrong a 50-metre head start in the 100-metre dash.

There had been many first days of my menstrual cycle before this one, when I would begin cramping and, knowing my period was on the way, curse it. But this first day was different. It was exciting. The cycle-monitoring protocol was front and centre on the fridge. My first cycle under observation unfolded as expected, and by Day 12 there was a follicle ripe for insemination. Chad provided a sample, which then went into the sperm cocktail shaker with his most improved sperms.

In the exam room, I was given my undressing instructions. Dr. Silver Fox marched into the procedure room, armed with a catheter of what he callously referred to as a "terrible sample." Rather than join the sperm shaming, I prayed for a miracle.

As I walked bravely out of the clinic doors, the tears started to gather, but I held them in. I shared the news with my husband and we rode home in silence, thinking our own thoughts. As our infertile egos deflated a little more, we learned the lesson that assisted reproductive treatment isn't a perfect science.

When you first begin assisted fertility treatment, you are confident that it will produce a child. First, and primarily, science is a trusted discipline. Second, you are paying for treatment; it is expensive, and there is a no-refund policy. Last, you believe your body won't fail you, especially after you have spent time, money, and energy fertilizing your soil. But with failed cycle after failed cycle, you realize that you have a fucking infertility problem that even science, money, and hope can't fix.

After a handful of failed intrauterine inseminations, we decide to change protocols and shift our treatment focus to in vitro fertilization (IVF), which meant upping the baby-making ante by injecting myself with needles full of synthetic hormones to make my ovaries bloat with follicle overload. We began in July 2013. While I was excited about the possibility of having a baby via IVF, I was not looking forward to injecting my abdomen daily. Throughout the cycle, I excused myself from social invitations. I needed to stay focused and direct my energy to growing my sweet baby follicles.

The stimulation cycle of IVF went well; my cycle-monitoring days were uneventful. My blood work showed steadily increasing hormones, and by the fourth ultrasound, my follicles were ready to harvest. The retrieval was an experience. The procedure room was sterile and cold, and the line-up of medical practitioners made us uncomfortable. From the back, Chad observed the anaesthesiologist step forward to collect his $300 fee before injecting my IV with drugs that knocked me out. While I slept, the medical staff used a giant needle to magically pluck eggs from my ovaries and handed them over to the lab technicians. I woke up in the recovery room. The nurse coordinator told me that she helped me get dressed while Chad was busy contributing to his end of the baby-making bargain. I felt embarrassed knowing that I'd been naked in front of so many strangers.

Within the hour, we headed home knowing we had 10 good follicles to fertilize.

The next day the lab called with the news that my 10 good follicles were reduced to 5 embryos. By Day 5, we had three excellent blastocysts; we transferred one embryo and froze its two blastocyst siblings for later. The post-embryo-transfer instructions were simple: minimal activity for 24 hours. The two-week wait after IVF was treacherous: the progesterone suppositories intensified the abdomen twinges, back acne, and mood swings. Ten days after the fresh-embryo transfer, I attributed the spotting I was having to implantation bleeding. By noon that day, I had stopped calling it implantation bleeding and called it Day 1, the start of my menstrual cycle. The clinic later confirmed that the transfer had been unsuccessful, as my pregnancy-test blood work returned a big fat negative.

There were not enough tissues to dry my eyes. I felt like a barren woman who would never conceive. While we wallowed in our tears, sadness, and pity, we packed our bags for a weekend away in the city. My brother was getting married and we were both in the wedding party. Luckily, with enough cold alcoholic beverages, we were in good enough spirits to celebrate.

After the failed transfer, my perfectionist personality kicked it up a notch. While our doctor thought one failed cycle was acceptable, I disagreed. I was sensing a bigger-picture problem. Refusal to fail was ingrained in my DNA, so I continued my search for someone to help me fix my damn infertility problem. My search engine skills brought me to a fertility-specific acupuncturist. At our first appointment, I repeated the facts of our so-called infertile life and explained the outcome of the treatments we had tried. Her protocol included daily Chinese tea and herbs and weekly appointments to rebalance my *qi* and restore my vital fertile energy to help me get pregnant. I purchased the deluxe acupuncture package that cost close to $1,000.

Next, I welcomed a second naturopathic doctor to my team. Her focus was on women's health and infertility of all types. At our first appointment, she discussed her own struggle to conceive and told me she now had three children. A sucker for winning, I agreed to add more expensive fertility-boosting vitamins to my diet and future visits to my calendar. Between work, fertility-boosting appointments, and the rest of my life, I'd scheduled myself to the max. It felt like my brain was working on autopilot. I just kept on keeping on.

Rolling into the fall of 2013, I felt confident about the upcoming frozen-embryo transfer. Over the previous eight weeks, I'd been following a supercharged fertility regiment chock full of Zen-like activities, such as acupuncture, yoga, and drinking Chinese tea. The cycle monitoring unravelled normally. My lining could have been thicker, but it was average. Transfer day arrived without a hitch and I straddled the embryo-transfer saddle. The masked lady opened the secret door from the lab and passed the fully loaded catheter to the administering doctor, who then shot me up with my own embryo. The two-week wait was atrocious; my mind raced with competing thoughts. Sometimes I thought I was pregnant, but other times I thought I was just going crazy. Post-transfer, I ate only warm, cooked foods, I played the embryo music, I binge watched Netflix, and I prayed.

November 1, 2013: pregnancy blood-test day. With the first transfer, my menstrual cycle had started before my pregnancy-test results were in. But with this transfer, there was no sign of my period. Our emotions were in limbo as we waited anxiously by our phones for the clinic's notification. By noon, an email had arrived in my inbox from the nurse coordinator. It sadly confirmed my second negative pregnancy-test result. I hung my head in frustration.

I was not happy with how my life was turning out. I retreated into a quiet headspace. On the outside I appeared brave, but I was weak. Since the beginning of our growing fertility concerns, Chad and I had not wanted the pity of others. We had enough of our own to wallow in. We tried not to be the couple who enters a room looking emotionally haggard. But to do that, we needed some quiet time to regroup. It became difficult to motivate myself to celebrate someone else's happy. But we did the best we could for the ones we loved. By this point, I felt the toll this was all taking on my well-being, and I just wanted this emotional nightmare to end.

At the next appointment at the clinic, we discussed alternative treatment options. Without an exact diagnosis for our infertility, I found it difficult to comprehend what the fuck was going on. We had problem-solved to the *nth* degree and still had no solution to our so-called infertile life. We questioned Dr. Silver Fox. Should I continue to try or should we change the game plan? We discussed our options in their entirety and left our appointment feeling dazed. Neither of us could believe our shitty luck in our quest to be parents. As young, healthy, and physically fit adults, it was difficult for us to digest the magnitude of our reproductive failures, and we questioned why our bodies would fail us in this way.

With another new year around the corner, we forced ourselves to think positive thoughts — until my newly married younger brother announced they were expecting. I'm sure that my initial reaction was the exact opposite of the majority of reactions they received. But after the year I'd had, I just needed them and their happiness to go away. I understood how my less-than-celebratory reaction hurt their feelings, but it was nothing personal or intentional. It was just that I could feel my once-happy life slipping through my fingertips and myself coming undone. What I needed was for someone in my life to take a minute and empathize with my broken heart. I was not just having a bad day; I was repeatedly having bad years. My experience with reproductive treatment was never something I could simply explain to friends. Only those who had struggled to conceive could truly understand my sorrow. It was during these times I realized that my heart would always ache if I didn't have someone to call me Mom.

Midway into 2014, we prepared for our final frozen-embryo transfer. I was cautiously optimistic that the third time would be a charm. The two-week waiting period was an all-too-familiar experience: treacherous, internet consuming, and confusing. I was no longer fascinated by the mantra of pregnant until proven otherwise.

With the news that the third transfer was not a success, it felt like my fate had been sealed. I was absolutely confident that we'd tried everything within reason to get pregnant. If there was a vitamin, we had consumed it; an alternative medicine health practitioner, we had tried them; a book, we had read it; a magic potion, we had drunk it. But still no baby. To date, we'd spent over $20,000 on fertility treatments, and the burden of it all was drowning our marriage.

With no more embryos to transfer, we had to decide on either a full stop to the baby-growing business or a second round of hormone-injecting IVF. This was a difficult conversation between us because we hadn't ever considered not having children and we certainly hadn't considered spending $40,000 trying. While most of our married friends were enjoying their marital bliss and welcoming children into their lives, it felt like our infertility was casting doubt on our commitment to our vows. We did our best to never blame each other, we kept talking, and we worked together.

During difficult times, we grew distant with friends because we needed our space. Saying no to social celebrations allowed us to quietly sort through our emotions. In our circle, our infertility updates quickly moved to the back burner. We didn't care to chat about the hormones, needles, treatments, finances, or grief anymore. I had no more tears to cry when I explained why we had no baby five years into our marriage.

I was tired of feeling like a failure and I wanted off this emotional roller coaster. I took to the internet to research alternatives to bearing a child and read about surrogacy, embryo adoption, sperm and egg donors, and private adoption. As we learned the basics involved for each, we were able to prioritize our options. We reasoned that embryo adoption and genetic material donations were strategies for a later day. We agreed to search out surrogacy in Ontario. I learned that the websites of most clinics that facilitate these complex relationships provided a brief view of shared biographies, successes, and candidates in waiting. Women within my circle of friends and family volunteered to carry our child, but they were either pregnant or had dusty, cobwebby uteruses. It wasn't until we had a conversation with Chad's sister that we realized we might have found "the one." She was above the prime age for fertility, but she was a blessed mom of four and I trusted her.

But first we agreed to a second round of IVF with additional testing of the embryos' genetic material. This would help us rule out abnormalities for past and future purposes. The genetic testing was an additional $3,500 U.S. It was never the irrational amount of money we were spending on reproductive medicine that scared me. What scared me was that I was not ready to accept the possibility of a childless marriage.

The second round of IVF proved just as fun as the first. The hormone-induced stimulation and retrieval went as expected. The days before retrieval required stretchy, high-waisted pants because I was bloated and uncomfortable. My cycle produced 17 follicles with four good-looking blastocysts, which were biopsied and put on ice. The waiting period from freezing to genetic-test result day was three weeks. We were so conditioned to hearing bad news that when the doctor confirmed all four embryos were chromosomally normal, I cried. My heart healed just a little. We'd been abnormal too often, so this news of normal embryos felt refreshing.

Chad and I did some soul searching over the kitchen table. We asked each other questions that challenged our mental, emotional, and physical selves. We were honest with each other and shared our desires and needs for growing our family. Before we made a decision about what to do with our four normal embryos, we had to be on the same page about how we should move forward with our treatment options. We both had to be able to support the other's fertility failures and embrace moving on.

Chad and I decided we wanted the embryos to have the best chance at life. We decided to try with a gestational surrogate. Without doubt, I had given everything to my body trying to conceive. Maybe I had tried too much or too hard; maybe if I had relaxed a little it would've magically happened, but I had done it the way I needed to. I grew to believe that I didn't have to be pregnant to build my dreams of family. During the process of forgiving my uterus, I realized that recapturing my emotional self needed to be a priority. I wanted my life, my marriage, and my happy back. So, with cautious optimism, we bravely reached out to the most amazing woman we know.

In the fall of 2014, we welcomed my husband's sister, Beth, to the Baby Armstrong Problem-Solving Team. She had done some soul searching of her own to come to the decision to help us build our family. Her husband and four children were supportive and encouraged her to fulfill the role we were asking her to play. I asked if she was sure about this a thousand times, and a thousand times her confidence never waivered. She was the perfect surrogate: her family was complete, her children were budding independent teenagers, and she was kind and unbelievably selfless.

There were quite a few boxes we had to tick off before proceeding with a frozen-embryo transfer using a gestational surrogate. We checked the first box after Dr. Silver Fox approved her physical health to carry a child. Her above-average age for fertile success was of no concern, and we had no reason to doubt her fertile capabilities.

The second box required a passing grade on our mental health. On paper, this sounds like a necessary measure, but it isn't too difficult a test to pass. The clinic assigned a mental-wellness assessor, who required separate meetings with each couple. We needed her professional validation that we were entering this relationship having considered the variables and the consequences without coercion. In our session, we discuss a broad range of topics designed to test our emotional stability and how we really felt about having a gestational carrier. She dug into our past, present, and future. What concerned us was her uninformed curiosity about how we planned to tell a child born from this arrangement that they had a birth mother and a biological mother. I began to wonder if this assigned practitioner had even read through my medical file. As if we had thought that far ahead.

We were zero for three in bringing life to our embryos, on top of more than two years of other failed treatment protocols. For my own well-being, I had stopped thinking about baby names and nursery decor long ago. So we didn't have an answer to her question. But we agreed that should a child be born using a gestational carrier, we would figure out the best way to not confuse said child with their birth story. She told us that it would be the pregnant surrogate who received the glory and attention while the baby was in utero, but come birth, it would be the new parents who received the love and affection with baby in arms. What we took away from our mental-health session was that we had to fully come to terms with the reality of the situation and that there would be many emotional and mental challenges ahead.

The final box we had to tick included securing the legally binding intricacies of the relationship between a gestational carrier and the intended parents. This was a necessary formality to protect everyone's legal rights and interests. Should our child be born to my husband's sister, we had to make sure each party's parental declarations were in writing. We were only mildly prepared for the first appointment with our fertility lawyer. We spent a full evening being bombarded with questions we had never imagined having to answer: "Should you die, who is the guardian of your embryos? If your surrogate is brain dead, do you want her to be kept alive until her body can deliver the baby?" These were painful questions because they evoked both selfish and selfless emotional responses. We needed time to think about some of the more difficult ones.

From an intended parent's perspective, the exercise of structuring and following through with the legal agreement of renting a womb was exhausting and humiliating. The legal procedures were unempathetic, outdated, and expensive. The formalness of the situation hit us between the eyes, and the beautiful gift we were being given was soured by paperwork, DNA testing, and court dates. We absolutely understood the necessity of clearly agreed-upon parental declarations, but with the growth of privatized, modern reproductive medicine helping more and more couples to conceive, we felt that the legal approach to facilitating these relationships could be less gruelling.

We were fortunate that when we relayed the message of how the whole womb rental agreement worked, Beth and her husband nodded their heads, all in. We agreed to navigate the formal obstacles the best we could. We expected some bumps and bruises to our egos as we worked out the black and white, but we agreed to build this relationship with open communication. My overactive brain must have overwhelmed my calm, cool, and collected sister-in-law as I flooded her inbox with information I learned at appointments with doctors, naturopaths, and lawyers and as I researched the best foods for fertility. My Type-A brain didn't need to know what she did with the emails; she could have deleted them or she could have added a few ideas to her grocery list. I just needed to participate in the relationship we were growing.

In the spring of 2015, we transferred one frozen embryo into our gestational surrogate. Her uterine lining was far better looking than mine. For a mature-aged woman, her cycle was textbook perfect. During the all-life-consuming cycle monitoring, I tried to compensate her for the time and energy she was devoting to something important to me. We reimbursed her for out-of-pocket expenses and supplied her with prenatal basics and were quiet cheerleaders from the sidelines.

The medical chart no longer had my name on it. It takes confidence in yourself to hear another woman's name being called for your embryo transfer. I was no longer an active participant in the baby-making game. I decided not to join the medical team in the transfer room. I knew what to expect, and my sister-in-law deserved her privacy.

With the embryo transfer complete, we kept Beth cooped up for 36 hours so she could rest, and then we kindly returned her to her own family. Chad and I helped out around her house and with her children in hopes that this already busy wife and mother could spare a fraction of energy to grow our embryo into a baby. Before we let her be, I prepared a week's worth of precooked meals for her freezer and packed the pantry with healthy snacks: nuts, seeds, and gluten-free oatmeal. During the two-week wait to see if the embryo nested in nicely, we spent quite a bit of time together. I thought I was doing a good job of giving her some privacy and space, but I hadn't been given a how-to guide for my new position on the Baby Armstrong Team. I was learning how to be an "intended mother" as we went along. I had to retrain my brain to hand over control of how she would be pregnant with my child. Her fertility track record and patient personality encouraged me to trust her.

Late in the morning before our pregnancy blood test, Beth sent us a video message that ended with a picture of a home pregnancy test with double pink lines. We immediately called her and exchanged tears of joy. To be sure, we kept asking her questions. Did she pee on the test stick right? How long did she hold it in the urine stream? But, confident she knew how to take a home pregnancy test, we allowed ourselves to believe in this happy ending.

The next day, a warm spring day, Beth, my mother-in-law, and I sat on the front porch, casually gabbing about the possibility of a baby and waiting for the clinic to send a confirmed-pregnancy email. As Beth read the clinic's news of a low hCG level aloud, I read between the lines. Her low level of human growth hormone likely indicated a pregnancy that would fail to thrive. Tears stung my eyes, but I didn't let them fall. I wouldn't let Beth see my sadness. She was almost pregnant, and she had to believe good things could still happen. After the repeat test, a chemical pregnancy was confirmed. Her hCG had not doubled; it had dropped. She was given permission to stop progesterone, and her menstrual cycle would arrive in due time. As I hung my head in utter frustration, I reflected on how good it had felt to let down my emotional guard and almost feel happy. Our families grieved for our almost happy ending. In the weeks that followed, we respected each other's privacy and grieved the loss we so intimately shared.

Midway through the summer of 2015, we brought to the table the conversation of whether Beth and her family were willing to try a second embryo transfer. We were prepared for her to change her mind. We absolutely would have understood if the time, energy, and emotional investment were just too much for her and her family. But they embraced the storm we weathered, and as a family they willingly agreed to a second embryo transfer. We sighed with relief and, sitting together around their kitchen table, we relaxed our tired minds with a bottle of wine. We found comfort in the relief of having someone to share our so-called infertile life with. After a few glasses of wine, it was easier for me to push the envelope on how we would approach the next transfer. Wincing, I said that we would like to try adding a few more prenatal supplements to boost her fertile ingredients and ask her to stop caffeinating. This family loves their coffee, so I knew it was a big request. Knowing I had good intentions, she patiently entertained my desperate, hyper-focused brain.

To hand over the reins of control wasn't easy. I had to accept that she wasn't always going to do things my way. Not because she didn't love me, but because she was her own person with her own control panel. She had her own job, life, and family, along with her own responsibilities and routines. Without a doubt, there were surely times she wanted to throw me and my frozen protein shakes and precooked meals out her door. But she didn't ever make us feel like we were infringing on her life. She reassured me that, within reason, she would do whatever was best for baby.

In the late summer of 2015, we were set to attempt a second frozen-embryo transfer. It had been a summer of strengthening the relationship between our families. My family reached out to Beth's family, got to know them, and showed their appreciation for their kindness. As a family, we spent a lot of time together, driving to and from appointments, talking over lunches, laughing over the phone, and building relationships. There haven't been too many relationships in my life that have made me feel as grateful or loved.

Days before the scheduled transfer, my husband's grandfather passed away. Gramps was a man my husband and Beth held dear to their hearts. Selfishly, the thread of doubt unwound my mind and I wondered if Beth's emotional state was going to be the right temperature for getting pregnant.

I told her that if in any way she felt too sad, I would prefer to wait until she felt happier. But she and her family encouraged us to continue. They were all in good enough places with the passing of their patriarch. So we moved forward with the transfer.

After the transfer, we shuttled our pregnant-until-proven-otherwise surrogate home, where we prepared warm, nourishing meals. We got her cozy in the recliner with Netflix and implantation-friendly snacks. We passed time reflecting on life and how maybe Gramps had to pass to give life to new family. It felt overly hopeful to believe in the idea of taking life to give life, but in desperation we held on to this belief. The week following the transfer, both families helped look after Beth's children and her household so she could relax knowing her family was taken care of while she busied herself taking care of ours.

This was our fifth frozen-embryo transfer and quite possibly the last. The two-week wait to see if I would be a mother was, again, torturous, and my mind and emotions were on the fritz. Almost a hundred times a day, I wanted to ask Beth if she was having any twinges, cramping, or nausea, but following my better judgment, I didn't. I ticked the days off and filled my social calendar with anything to distract me: lunches, shopping, DIY projects. On pregnancy-test day, there were no positive feelings pulsing through my body. We asked Beth that if she took a home pregnancy test, she not share any news with us prior to the clinic's email with confirmed blood test results.

We checked our email accounts 900 times a minute until the message finally appeared at midday. We nervously opened the email and saw an animated flying stork and the words "Congratulations. Your pregnancy test is positive with an hCG value of three hundred and five." I hugged my husband and sobbed on his shoulder. We both exhaled stale breath and called our confirmed-pregnant goddess. We swapped happy tears and baby-mama jokes. Wide-eyed with disbelief, we reread the email to enjoy the moment again.

Our families were eager to celebrate the growth of our family in 2016. But before we announced our news, Chad and I needed some time to adjust to the reality of the circumstances. In the last five years, we had poured every ounce of our time, energy, money, love, and hope into a confirmed pregnancy, and today here it was. I marked up the calendar with the latest schedule of ultrasounds, blood work, and all things leading to a viable pregnancy.

The happy thoughts faded away once the reality of waiting for the seven-week viability scan set in. My compulsion to forecast the what-ifs of this early pregnancy strangled my thought process. I wasted my time researching catastrophes.

Chad and I decided that during this pre-viability waiting period, we needed to refocus our energy, so we packed our bags and got out of town. We love New York City for all its distracting lights, people, and noise. We booked a hotel in the fashion district and made reservations for new dining experiences and a Broadway show. It was fall, so it was rainy and cool. We walked aimlessly throughout the city, window shopping, café hopping, and swaying through Central Park, flipping coins into every wishing well we passed. As we sipped daytime beers and drank evening wine, we let go of some negative inhibitions. We talked about life as we knew it and the possibility of change, and we continued to forgive each other for our fertility failures. We recommitted to our marriage, children or not, and bravely held on to the hope that next week we would be introduced to our baby.

The following week, Chad and I anxiously waited with the other expecting fathers in the ultrasound department. Beth was in the exam room, and I, the biological mother, was not allowed in for the initial procedure. The news of my baby's viability would come second-hand. This was just one of many insulting aspects of being "just" the intended mother. Every time an exam room door opened or closed, my heart skipped a beat. I was sweating and holding my breath. After approximately 45 minutes, Beth appeared around the corner and waved us in. My heart dropped as I contemplated why she would be coming to call us in. Shouldn't she be waiting on the exam table, ready to show us our baby? As I entered without waiting for pleasantries, I scanned the dark room. I looked from the ultrasound tech to the monitor to Beth and nervously asked if there was a baby. Beth smiled widely and I could feel my heart heal, just a little. With tears welling in my eyes, I hugged everyone in the room, the crying tech included. Together, we rewound the video replay and I watched and listened to my baby's tiny heart palpitating, fighting for life.

As the first trimester trickled along, I downloaded a baby-development app and watched our baby grow from a kidney bean to a pea pod. Between the early viability scan and our 13-week ultrasound, our little one began to look less like a baby dinosaur and more like a baby human. Week after week, I checked the app to see how the baby was developing. I learned to use the power of thought to connect to my unborn child. I appreciated the information available via the internet because, as an intended mother, I could only learn second-hand how my baby was doing. I was not the patient and, therefore, due to the legalities of patient confidentiality, unless Beth was present, I could not access information about my child. This fact took some getting used to because it was emotionally insulting to my idea of motherhood.

As one trimester turned into two, my husband and I allowed ourselves to outwardly embrace another woman bringing our child into the world. I didn't want to buy the book to guide me on how to be an intended mother, because the more I read, the more pressure I put on myself to fix, change, or try harder. I had to teach myself to let go of the negative thoughts I had about my infertility and embrace the opportunity I had been given. We shared our baby-mama drama with friends, colleagues, health professionals, and nosy sales clerks. Some shared overly opinionated facial expressions, some considered us a social experiment, but most warmly accepted the news of our growing family with tears and celebratory hugs. Every one of my immediate friends and family supported our pursuit of family. Of course, there were instances where we encountered judgment, ignorance, and humiliation because of our infertility. But these experiences taught me about my own resilience and strengthened my ability to let go of the negative thoughts I had about myself. With time, I learned to love how the story of my life was unfolding.

At the baby's anatomy scan, Chad and I didn't want to be told the baby's gender among the crowd of people there. Beth's husband and children were joining us at this ultrasound appointment. We all believed it was important to introduce everyone and encourage them to participate in building this relationship. Beth's husband and three sons were supportive and excited to meet their youngest cousin. The tech was kind and recognized our need to learn our baby's gender privately. We left with a sealed envelope.

Beth's baby bump started to grow and I tried not to physically hover over her belly. I craved some private time with my baby. I wanted to nurture it, to feel it kick, move, hiccup, and induce nausea. I was counting the days until I could physically hold and bond with my child. I had to settle for texts with daily updates and video replay of baby kicking across her stomach. When I was in Beth's presence, I had to be mindful of how physical and emotional I was with the baby. I realized that we were both sorting through different emotions, thoughts, and feelings. While I was trying to nest and prepare for the baby by buying all the things new moms need, such as car seats, strollers, diapers, and newborn-size onesies, she was preparing to relinquish the life growing inside her. There was no one to teach me how to watch another woman grow my child, and there was no one to teach her how to compartmentalize the love she had for the child growing inside of her. We were both the child's life-givers, and regardless of who was carrying the baby or who shared the biology, we fell in love. We were fortunate that between us, we had a great support team who constantly checked in with our preparedness and made sure we were acknowledging and coping with how this fairy tale would end.

As we counted down the weeks to the third trimester, our anticipation to know our unborn child built. Sometime after the 25-week mark, I let my emotional guard down. With time, I started to heal, and each time I shared my story I grew prouder of us for not giving up. During the five years of our so-called infertile life, my husband and I had encountered many opportunities to blame each other and walk away from our commitment. But we had both held on to the hope that one day we would be parents and enjoy the beauty of loving a child together.

One weekday evening Chad and I headed out for dinner, sealed envelope in hand. We were fast approaching the third trimester, and it was time we let ourselves feel like expecting parents. It was time to let our hearts in on what our minds already knew. Over a celebratory pasta dinner we fell wildly in love reading the big bold print: "IT'S A BOY!!!!!!" We both gasped in awe. A son, growing day by day in preparation of our first embrace.

Chad and I kept the gender of our unborn child between us a little longer. We craved the privacy; our fertile laundry had been airing long enough. We allowed ourselves to shop for our baby boy, plan his nursery, and start saying his name out loud. By the 30-week mark, I could feel the happy returning to my life.

Early in our expecting journey, I had decided I didn't want a baby shower. I was obviously not pregnant, and I didn't know how I felt about celebrating another woman's womb. However, the women in my life thought it was important that we celebrate the beauty of the experience, and I eventually agreed. What I learned at the shower was that the women were there to celebrate motherhood, womanhood, and my courage to share my story. Through different conversations I was able to open up to these women, sharing how discouraging our infertility had been. I did my best to openly thank Beth for being my greatest advocate and for gifting me the miracle of life. As I willingly shared my emotions, there was not a dry eye in the room. I could see that each of these women was identifying with my grief. Some were thinking about their love for their own children, some were thinking about their own losses, and some were grieving the children they were unable to conceive. The hugs we exchanged lasted a little longer than usual. I realized these women were proud of me, and we celebrated not just the baby, but the beauty of kindness, love, and supporting the women in our lives.

Our son unexpectedly made his arrival two weeks early, four days after the baby shower, and we were unprepared. The night he decided to make his presence known, we were out for dinner with friends, enjoying a gourmet meal and celebrating with bottles of wine. We toasted our last pre-baby dinner. Once home, we had just nestled into bed when the phone rang.

On May 5, 2016, at 10:30 p.m., Beth's water broke. Despite living two hours away, she wanted to make the drive to Markham Stouffville Hospital, where we were preregistered. Realization set in, then panic. There was no hospital bag packed. My SUV with the newborn carrier and car seat was at the dealership for repair. I had no sterilized bottles, no formula, and no cute newborn outfit picked out. The irony of my lack of preparation, when throughout this whole thing I had been nothing but prepared, was not lost on me. I called my sister and she tried to list off the necessities I would need to bring with us to the hospital. I thought I was in shock.

Well past midnight, we were admitted to the labour and delivery unit. The medical staff on shift immediately responded to and accommodated both the birthing and the biological parents. We were all shown empathy and respect by these medical professionals. They involved Chad and me in the birthing process; we were given hospital bracelets and hospital gowns and, for the first time, we were made to feel like every expecting parent feels when they are about to deliver a baby.

The delivery doctor encouraged me to participate in the birth of my son. She was assertive and literally pulled my hands into position to catch and welcome him into the world. After a quick wipe down, he was placed into my open arms and I whispered, "It was you." I told him that it was his heart that I had heard calling my name; it was his face I had seen smiling in the ultrasound; it was he who had chosen me.

Chad participated like every new dad. He cut the umbilical cord, hung over the nurse as she assessed the baby's birth score, and recorded the birth details. After Beth had been taken care of by the nurses, her arms were next in line so she could hold the baby and introduce herself.

After the delivery, we spent some private time together before introducing our son to his anxiously waiting grandparents, aunts, uncles, and cousins. As he was passed around the room, love was exploding from everyone's hearts as we were all reminded that miracles do happen. This little guy had a birth story that was complicated but beautiful. For us, his life would serve as a reminder to be the best people we could be to ourselves and to others.

I lost five good years to my so-called infertile life. My struggle to conceive changed me. I no longer force myself to be perfect; I realize that I'm happy being perfectly imperfect. I now make a consistent effort to check in with the people in my life. I care more about how they are doing. I care less about materialistic things and more about just being happy with myself and my life story. Of course, my Type-A brain continues to micromanage the domestic doings of our household. But I have learned to let go. I no longer think that I'm entitled to a picture-perfect life. I now know that no matter how much I try, some things just don't work out as planned, and that's okay. After my parental leave, I chose to reduce the juggling in my life. I have fought hard to be a mom and I want to give my family my best. I want to give my life's miracle as much time and love and as many hugs as I can before he starts squirming away from my reach. I lost out on the opportunity to physically bond with my child in utero, so we are constantly making up for lost time.

Despite welcoming a son in a way we never imagined, the love we share for *us* outweighs the importance of how he arrived into our lives. My husband and I fought hard for him and we will never let him forget it. I now choose to look on the bright side of my struggle to conceive and my son's life story. The struggle was real, and it taught me many valuable and humbling lessons about self-entitlement and taking things for granted. As a result, I'm a more grateful wife, a more loving mother, and a more supportive friend. I now take time to smell the roses and do things that are important to me. So, while I will never thank my infertility outright for the unhappiness it caused me, I can appreciate it for what it taught me about myself and the kind of life I want for my family.

There will never be enough gifts, hugs, or praise to show my sister-in-law how amazing I think she is. Her selfless perspective on helping others is one in a million. In return, she only asks that we always love our son unconditionally.

Now that I have someone calling me Mama, I have my happy back. My once-broken heart is overflowing with love for my son, whether he giggles, cries, plays, or sleeps. My husband and I are continually reminded of how lucky we are to have our son, and we often remind each other of how happy we are to finally move on from our so-called infertile life.

1 2
18 EGGS

Cynthia Cyr

I'M PRETTY SURE MY HUSBAND, Marty, has autism spectrum disorder. I'm not a doctor, and he's never been properly diagnosed, but I worked in social services for nearly five years with many people across the autism spectrum, and he definitely displays some of the telltale signs.

For example, he rarely makes eye contact with anyone, even me. I think he's paying attention when we're talking, but I can't tell for sure. Also, he doesn't notice when I walk in or out of a room, even if it's just the two of us. His observance of the atmosphere doesn't change; he continues to read or play games on his iPad without interruption. I've watched him take command of a complicated business discussion, wondering how he can be so in tune with so many people at once, yet not realize when I need him unless I specifically tell him what I need him for. I catch him repeating the name of our recently deceased dog over and over again under his breath, almost every single day. I never say anything about it to him, even though it fills my guts with sadness. I know that, however weird his behaviour may be, this is how he has to work through the same heartbreak I'm going through.

His aloofness is often funny and endearing in social settings. More than once, I've been told I should write a show about Marty, or pitch a reality show where he's followed around by cameras. But that's how he is only some of the time; the Marty I share with our social network. Sometimes — actually, a lot of the time — when we are alone together, my

Marty comes off as cold and apathetic. I have to put double the amount of warmth into our relationship in an effort to ensure that we, at the very least, maintain some kind of neutrality. Sometimes I don't have the extra 100 percent in me to give.

But there are moments of tenderness that mean so much more to me than they would from any other person, since they are so few and far between. I can think of no other person I would want on my side in an emergency. We are almost always on the same page when it comes to making joint decisions. He has planned surprise visits and trips for my best friends to come see me when I feel lonely. He's by far the strangest person I know, and I love him times a millionfinity.

This story isn't about Marty, although I know it's a weird opening to say that only now. This story is about our struggle with infertility. Given that I'm the one narrating, I think it's only fair you understand why he plays such a minor role in our collective story.

Before we got married, we discussed having children. Not in a let's-sit-down-and-plan-our-future serious way, but in the way that many young people growing up in a small town do. We understood marriage and children to be the main courses of adulthood. We were both on board for careers, marriage, purchasing a home, and one child. Neither of us was interested in starting a family immediately, and we agreed that one would be enough for us.

We hit a bit of a roadblock when it came to purchasing a home. We were living in Toronto and found ourselves caught in several bidding wars. Unable to secure something that worked for us, we decided to take a break from house hunting and invested our resources in adventures instead. We travelled around the world, attended outdoor music festivals, and partied into early mornings. We camped in the Sahara Desert, chatting with friends under the stars. We had years of magical, carefree living.

During our third year of marriage, we made the decision to move to Vancouver. Marty was offered a business expansion opportunity with his firm, and I jumped at the chance to start another new adventure. We packed a rental car with very few things and our giant, slobbering dog, Taiko, and drove across the country toward our new life.

It was a hard move for me. In Toronto, we had had many friends and were close enough to Ottawa, our hometown, so we could visit family. I enjoyed my job as an advertising producer and I liked the people I worked with. I was always so busy and I loved it. In my head, I imagined our new life would be much like our life in Toronto, just by the ocean. Although I quickly found a great new job at an amazing agency, we knew very few people in Vancouver. The time difference made it difficult to connect with family and friends back home, and it turns out that I'm not really that outdoorsy. Now that I'm well-adjusted to this beautiful city, I can't imagine not living here, but I harboured feelings of disdain those first few years.

Marty loved Vancouver immediately. He didn't need friends or family close by or to be entertained in the same way I did. His business was thriving. Even Taiko, who always seemed like an old dog, acted five years younger. I searched online for the "most beautiful loft in Vancouver" and told Marty I wanted to live there. He said okay and we moved in soon after. It should have been enough for me.

At this point, most of my friends were raising their second child, and although I didn't want more than one, it felt like the right time to at least start the conversation with Marty. On the flip side, some of my other girlfriends were experiencing difficulty getting pregnant, and Google worried me with articles about the early 30s being the beginning of declining fertility.

"Okay, I want to have a baby now," I declared over breakfast one day. I felt the air get sucked out of the room. The television sounded much louder all of a sudden as I watched his nonreaction for what seemed like a full minute. It was, to say the least, awkward, and not what I had anticipated. The obvious stall tactic leading up to a hesitant "I'm not sure it's the right time" response should have been a signal for what was to come.

I don't know why I was so confident. I'd never had a pregnancy scare. Not one. And I don't mean with Marty, whom I had been with for eight years by that point. I mean like ever, in my entire life. But my mom had had no issues getting pregnant, nor had my sister, and both of my parents come from huge families. I was sure it was going to be like this: step 1, sexy time; step 2, baby time. And they lived happily ever after.

When I didn't get pregnant right away, I did all the things the internet tells you to do. I tracked my cycle, did it in the "right" positions, dieted, exercised, and experimented with essential oils and crystals, whatever the old Google machine said would help. It gave me something to focus on while I was unhappy being so far from home. And if I am going to be completely honest, my head was in a weird "who needs home, I'll just grow my own family" kind of mentality. Trying was fun at first because it was new. Then, after a few months, it wasn't, because having sex with any goal in mind other than orgasm is the exact opposite of fun.

After about four months, I wanted to speak with a fertility specialist. Marty was against it at first; he was loving life as it was and didn't really want to disrupt the pattern. But I'd recently turned 35, and the pressure was definitely getting to me. I insisted that we at least have preliminary tests done to see if there was anything wrong with us.

As directed by my peers going through infertility treatment and by a handful of internet strangers, I lied and said we had been trying for a year, in order to expedite the initial consultation with the specialist. It came as a huge surprise when, during my initial patient evaluation, Dr. Kari explained that they did not consider pulling out to be a prevention method and made a note that we had actually been trying for the entire eight years we'd been together.

This was a very different situation than the pretend year I'd lied about. From there, things moved fast. Speaking with a fertility specialist quickly became committing to in vitro fertilization (IVF). Payments were requested; blood tests were scheduled; drugs were prescribed. It all went by in a blur. Marty only half paid attention, with the unspoken understanding that while he was green-lighting the funds, this was my project. We had both been on the fence for a while now, with him veering closer and closer to the no-baby zone and me still tottering around the middle. How do you successfully plan for a family when at least half of the decision-makers don't want to participate in the discussion?

We very rarely fight, but we fought a lot about this. I brought up past discussions where we had decided on raising a small family, silently accusing him of changing his mind, and he tried to get me to focus on the incredible life we had created together. Even still, we moved forward with the IVF process because I had tunnel vision and couldn't appreciate our life without constantly wondering what our other life could be like. I was left on my own to decipher the meaning of medical jargon and navigate unfamiliar corners of the Web, and the process felt lonely and stressful, particularly since I wasn't even sure if this was what I wanted or if I was persisting only because I wanted to be the boss of our marriage. While I appreciated the efficiency of the appointments and Dr. Kari's candid manner, I left every meeting with more questions than I had going in.

The main takeaway from our conversations with the specialist was that it was definitely an egg issue. Nothing came up as abnormal in karyotype, sperm, blood, or hysterosalpingogram tests. For some reason, this didn't surprise me at all. Of course, after all my insistence that we proceed with IVF, it would be my own body that kept me from moving forward.

Eventually, it became time to prep my body, meaning to stimulate follicle and ovaries. It was about a week of injections and oral medications and getting up at the crack of dawn for daily monitoring visits at the clinic. Between the drugs, lying to my work team about why I was constantly late in the mornings, and second-guessing everything about my life, the entire process made me feel like a crazy person. I got cold feet as the time to retrieve my eggs drew nearer. I still sort of wanted a baby, but I wasn't sure it was for the right reasons.

As I write this, nearly two years later, I know my reasons for wanting a baby weren't the right reasons, at least not for us. But back then, I ticked them off like items on a checklist: I wanted someone to take care of me when I was old, my friends were all having kids, it would be a great way to meet people in this new city … me, me, me. Now, while I know there isn't any single right reason to have a child, I think at least one of them should be that you want to be a parent, and this was glaringly absent from my list.

Instead of opting for the immediate embryo transfer that month, as originally planned, Marty and I discussed going through the cycle and then freezing the embryos for a later transfer date. We went over this with the IVF team and discovered the chances of a success with a frozen embryo were just as good as with a fresh one, and in some cases frozen embryos had even more potential. Our specialist discussed the option of transferring multiple embryos, explaining that the rate of success would increase and that we could potentially become pregnant with twins.

I didn't even have to do any research on that one. While some couples may see twins as a double blessing, or a two-for-one deal, all I could picture was two identical little girls with long dark hair and giant black eyes hovering over me when I woke up.

"Would you like some breakfast, Mother?" they would chant in unison. There would never be a breakfast.

Marty needed no convincing: there would be no multiple embryo transfers. We wanted a single frozen-embryo transfer sometime in the near future. We would let the clinic know when we wanted to do this a few months in advance. We would keep the remaining frozen embryos in case the single transfer was unsuccessful. The bills were stacking up, but I was proud of our grown-up decision-making and family planning. We could see from the ultrasound that I had developed a healthy number of mature eggs ripe for retrieval and there were no indications there would be any sort of complications with our plan.

Eighteen eggs were extracted from my body. Eighteen! We were all so confident then: me, Marty, my friends and family, the whole IVF team. I had expected 8 to 10 to be taken out, so 18 seemed incredible. My best friend had undergone the same process and only four eggs were extracted. I felt so lucky.

This was around the time the cockiness ended.

From there, the embryologist contacted me on a daily basis with a progress report, and it went something like this:

DAY 1: 9 OF 18 EGGS FERTILIZED

The results from the sperm wash were much lower than anticipated. The embryologist performed rescue intracytoplasmic sperm injection (ICSI), the process of selecting a single sperm from the semen sample and injecting it directly into the egg. She recommended freezing five-day blastocysts instead of the three-day embryos for a better chance of success.

But, like, nine fertilized eggs is still good, right? I mean, I had expected to have only around nine eggs retrieved in total. I swear I could hear pity in her voice when she explained that a 50 percent fertilization rate was actually not very good at all.

DAY 2: SIX EMBRYOS REMAINED

The embryologist experienced lower than anticipated results with the rescue ICSI, with only four of the remaining nine eggs being fertilized.

"That means I should have thirteen embryos in total, right? Including the nine from yesterday's ... haul?"

"Unfortunately, some of those embryos did not make it, so there are only six embryos in total that are currently viable," she said.

Are you a robot? I silently screamed at the top of my lungs. How was this even happening?

DAY 3: FOUR EMBRYOS REMAINED

More of the embryos were no longer viable, just like that. This would have been the day an embryo was supposed to be implanted into my uterus, so I felt weirdly sad, like I missed a birthday.

DAY 4: TWO EMBRYOS REMAINED

None of the embryos from the rescue ICSI were viable for freezing; the two remaining embryos were from the original sperm wash. This was supposed to be a good sign, that these two survived. That is what I was supposed to take away as good news after a week of being told we were experiencing lower than average results.

It was like watching some fucked-up fertility version of *The Hunger Games*, with my chances to reproduce dying off day by day. All I could do was wait for the final 24 hours to tick by and hope the two remaining embryos had some exceptional Katniss and Peeta survival story in the world I had created within my body as a reluctant game-maker. There's probably a better metaphor, but I was really into the series at the time. This was a long day of praying, which was weird because I'm not religious. I imagined raising twins named Katniss and Peeta and explaining to strangers that *The Hunger Games* played an extremely significant role in my life and I'm not just a weird grown-up fan lady.

It wasn't looking good, though. I used jokes to cope with having to explain the results to my inner circle, and no one needed to tell me the rate at which my embryos were being discarded was abnormally high.

DAY 5: ONE "JUST-OKAY" BLASTOCYST SURVIVED

The embryologist didn't say it like that, but she was thinking it — I just knew it. In fact, in my pent-up hormonal state after all of the fertility medication, I knew everyone was thinking it. The doctor, the receptionist,

Marty, my family and friends. Everyone. *How did she only produce 1 good embryo out of 18 eggs?* It wasn't even a super-good-quality one; it was just good enough to freeze. With the rate of success so far, I couldn't help but wonder if they just froze it for the sake of freezing something for us. A pity freeze because the procedure had cost upwards of $12,000.

I thought back to how confident Marty and I had been just one week before when we rejected the idea of implanting multiple embryos and how we were going to freeze "all the rest." We didn't even have the option anymore. I thought about those dark-haired girls with giant black eyes and cried and cried because they didn't look so scary anymore. They would have had the chubbiest faces, would have laughed a lot at their super-weird dad, and would never want to cut their hair, the same way I hadn't wanted to when I was young. And they would never exist now.

Dr. Kari sent over a nice email, asking us to come in to chat about the results.

"Certainly has the look of an egg issue this cycle," he began.

I had been told this numerous times throughout the process and I already felt defeated about it. I gritted my teeth and asked what could be done differently if we were to undergo another cycle. I was so fully blown up with emotions from the side effects of the medication and the crappy results of the IVF, I couldn't even tell whether I was considering another round (which we definitely couldn't afford) because I wanted to feel like my body wasn't a failure, or whether it was because I really wanted a successful pregnancy. As expected, Marty was only half present, checking his phone every few minutes. I almost left the room because I knew I wouldn't be able to fully remember all of the details in my emotionally elevated state and I needed him to listen. I kicked him under the table when Dr. Kari wasn't looking, and he loudly responded with an annoyed "What?" I quickly got embarrassed.

The doctor went into a few scenarios, but ultimately it sounded like guesswork to me. Often, the first cycle is more of a test for things like medication dosages. But I had produced 18 eggs with the provided dosage — the only higher than average results during my entire IVF process. It was the egg quality where I had an issue, not the quantity. What was wrong with my eggs?

Dr. Kari shrugged and said, "It could be a result of genes, it could be diet or smoking ... or other bad things you may have done to your body." His voice trailed off and he looked to his papers as if there was suddenly something really interesting there.

It was true, I had smoked cigarettes in my 20s. I still have a cigarette every now and then, but so few and far between that I never thought it would affect my fertility health. Almost everyone I know smokes sometimes, and most of my girlfriends, now in our early to mid-30s, are on their second children without any fertility complications.

But *other bad things* — I knew about those.

I have never really been a drinker, as a result of a terrible experience I had when I was a teenager and because of the ugly red blotches that appear on my body after a few sips. Alcohol tastes like nail polish remover to me, so I don't bother trying it anymore. Marty says, "I drink enough for the both of us" at pretty much every single social event we attend, and I am forever grateful for this small kindness disguised as a dad joke. He knows I hate explaining to strangers why I don't drink, because how do you politely explain that you don't like drunkenness and think alcohol tastes gross to someone who is about to imbibe? I wear this like a badge of honour, smugly declining offers of drinks at parties while keeping the jokes and good times flowing. "She doesn't drink, but she's cool."

Other bad things. The words ran over and over in my mind as if a terrible song I had forgotten about was now playing on repeat. The "Chumbawamba" of thoughts. Not drinking alcohol doesn't mean I've been a saint my whole life; I certainly spent enough time in my 20s in VIP, dancing through Sundays on speakers and solidifying new friendships while hovering over washroom toilets. I always conveniently leave that part out when I stoically wrinkle my nose at clumsy drinkers. Like smoking, I never thought casual use of designer drugs would affect me later in life. The bulk of my girlfriends had stopped partying because they got pregnant, whereas I stopped partying because I got bored of the scene. I never gave it a second thought, to be honest. Also, I met Marty around then, and the idea of him raging at the club is hilarious to me.

Were those bad things some 10 or 15 years ago the reason I couldn't get pregnant now? I'll never know, not for sure. So many thoughts ran through my mind: guilt weighing heavily for potentially ruining my body and my chances at motherhood with self-inflicted poisoning, coupled with visions of all the perfectly happy and healthy babies born to mothers who did the same things I did. Maybe a few of us undergo penance for everyone, and I was selected because I didn't care enough to pay attention. *I volunteer as tribute.* Okay, I'll stop with *The Hunger Games* now.

We decided to hold off on any further decision-making for a bit, Marty and I. He had made partner a few months earlier at his firm and wanted to take some time for us to absorb his new success and good fortune. We went to a nude resort in Nowhere, Mexico, where everything was hilarious because we were butt-naked doing mundane things, like asking where the pool towels were. We were very immature about it. We chased wildebeest from Kenya to Tanzania and went scuba diving in Zanzibar to find seahorses. We had the time of our lives experiencing the possibilities of life without children, and it was amazing. I travelled through Europe for a month, re-tracing steps from my early 20s and meeting up with some friends to sip cappuccinos and eat tapas late into the night. Life was so wonderfully easy with just us two, and I still found myself trying to feel something missing so I could clearly define space for a new addition.

We received a letter from the fertility clinic indicating our year lease was up on our frozen embryo's storage tank and we needed to pay a fee if we didn't want to move forward with the embryo transfer. A whole year had passed! It felt like it was just one second ago I was being probed and prodded regularly. I signed the letter and sent a cheque in the mail. I'm not ready. *We* aren't ready.

Our second-year lease will be coming down the pipe in a mere three months. Where did the time go? Marty rode a motorcycle through Japan. I quit my job and started my own business. Taiko died of cancer and our whole hearts were engulfed in mourning. It was a year of wonderful success coupled with crippling grief; there was no room to make family-planning decisions. Tick tock, tick tock. Even a non-decision eventually becomes a decision.

To be honest, I don't know if I'll ever be ready. People always respond by saying that no one is ever truly ready — you just have to go for it. But that's not really what I'm talking about when I say I'm not ready, although I have long since stopped correcting people. I understand now that it's gauche to say anything negative about raising a family, and doing so is likely to induce long pauses of discomfort. For others, it is always worth it; there is nothing more satisfying than having children.

But what if I physically can't do it? In addition to not being ready for parenting, I am also not ready to hear the words *the results were not as anticipated* for the umpteenth time about something I have zero control over but is still somehow my fault. For the sake of an annual $250, I find comfort in knowing our one embryo is safe in cryostorage, that its survival hasn't been risked by transferring it into my body. I only have about a 30 percent chance of a successful pregnancy with this single embryo, and if it fails, I have zero chances left. But as long as that single embryo is frozen in time, there's a good chance that future me will figure it out.

13

CIRCULAR INFERTILITY

Caroline Starr

WHEN I WAS 15, I had an irregular period.

When I was 16, I asked my mother if I could go on birth control. I wasn't yet having sex, but a lot of my friends were, and it seemed like the responsible thing to do. Even as a teenager, responsibility seeped out of me.

When I was 17, I became sexually active.

When I was 20, I forgot to pick up my birth control one month and decided to just skip the month and start another pack when I got my period.

When I was 21, I counted back and realized eight months had passed since I'd stopped taking birth control. I racked my brain to think whether there had been any opportunities for me to become pregnant. I realized I'd still been very responsible and careful, and it was unlikely. But I sent my boyfriend to buy a pregnancy test anyway, which would be the first of many tests to come back negative.

The doctor at my university's health services centre was very good looking, and it was uncomfortable for me to talk to him about nonexistent periods and my birth control experiment. I took another negative pregnancy test in the office. His uncertainty about what could be the cause was unsettling. I was referred to a large hospital and got an appointment with an obstetrician relatively fast. The quick referral made me feel like something about my condition was serious. These were the early days of the internet. Ask Jeeves was still the search engine of choice for many. I found very little information about what might cause someone to not have a period for the better part of a year. Things like cancer came up. By the time I had my specialist appointment, I was spinning with all the horrible possibilities of what could be wrong.

I brought my boyfriend with me to the appointment. He joined me, diligently, and listened along as a bunch of things, which I can't remember clearly, were checked, culminating in an uncomfortable internal ultrasound that showed my ovaries riddled with cysts.

"It's like a pearl necklace. That's what the condition is commonly called," the doctor said matter-of-factly, pointing to blurry white spots in a sea of fragmented black. "You have polycystic ovarian syndrome," also known as PCOS.

I was told that I needed to go back on birth control for PCOS maintenance and in order to have a regular period, and that if I wanted to have children, I shouldn't wait too long to start trying. I was told very little else.

At that point in my life, children were a far-off concept. I hadn't finished my undergraduate degree. My boyfriend and I were as serious as 21-year-olds could be, and we both liked kids well enough, but whether we were having them, let alone having them together, wasn't something we'd devoted a great deal of thought to.

One thing I've learned as a "proper" adult is that there's never time to process. Life is constantly hurled at you, and you spend so much time reacting that there's little time to mourn and grieve and process the big things. Life-changing things.

That appointment would change a lot for me. It would change the way I saw myself for the rest of my life. It would form the basis of my relationships with others.

That day, my boyfriend and I went back to work at our summer jobs immediately after the appointment.

Over the years that followed, we would occasionally discuss the future. I remember having a meltdown over infertility when we were teaching English in Japan when we were 22, and he told me it wasn't something we had to worry about right away. We would find a way. Or we could adopt. Everything would be fine. We'd figure it out.

I disagreed.

I spent a lot of time doubting his "we."

I said yes when Matt asked me to marry him a couple of years later.

Most of my 20s were spent on birth control, largely to keep my PCOS symptoms in check. On birth control, it was possible to maintain my weight and not get too hairy and have clockwork periods that I could predict by the hour. The other impacts, however, were less desirable, but because I'd been on it so long, I didn't realize until I went off it later that it had killed my sex drive and left me void of emotions and out of touch with my body.

Life marched on. We went to school for postgraduate stuff. We found jobs that turned into careers. We got a dog, followed by a cat. I continued to have infertility meltdowns every six months or so, and when I wasn't crying, I sat with this gnawing feeling in my gut that was so familiar I didn't realize it wasn't a normal or healthy way to feel.

I found myself in my late 20s, and the urgency to start a family increased, along with people asking when or if we were going to have children. Usually, it was accompanied by comments about what great parents we'd be, like framing something lovely in a piece of broken glass.

I saw doctors during this time. At least three. And had four or five internal ultrasounds. One doctor told me that I should get on an adoption list. When I was 26, a kindly Greek obstetrician nearing retirement told me after checking my insides that I'd have lots of babies. I carried his business card around for four years after that. As if it were proof I could haul out if anyone questioned me on fertility status. I had someone to refer to. This guy, with this office at Bloor and Sherbourne, said I'd be good. A bunch of people said I wouldn't be, but none of them knew as much as this guy.

Eventually, a time came when we decided that a kid was something we could manage. I was 28, and I stopped taking birth control the week we moved into our house, a milestone that had seemed impossible just a few years earlier. I felt okay about giving it a year and seeking intervention if it was required. I started setting aside money for fertility treatments instead of the kitchen renovation we wanted in our 100-year-old house with 1980s cabinets and peel-and-stick tiles on the floor.

I told myself it would be okay. That we'd waited, that we were here now, that we'd lived our lives, that now was the time. And that it would be okay.

When I went off birth control, I got my period after about 30 days. I took this to be a good sign.

My younger sister announced she was unexpectedly pregnant three weeks later.

It was hard to be happy for her.

We did our best to pretend it would just happen for us. I remember that trying in that first year was good. We had sex a lot. It was mostly enthusiastic. Eventually, though, when we hit 10 months, I gave in to the sinking feeling in my gut and went to see our family doctor.

I've been going to our doctor regularly for many years. We often disagree, but we're usually able to resolve our issues, and at the end of the day, he usually, as he says, treats the patient. When I showed up after 10 months and asked what we were doing wrong, he told me we needed to relax. He told us statistics that were supposed to be encouraging about the percentage of people who end up pregnant within a year. He said all the things that people said that weren't helpful.

I called him out on it.

He sheepishly offered to do a blood test to see if I'd ovulated that month, but told us we needed to try longer before he'd refer us to a clinic.

I had ovulated. So we were back to trying with renewed enthusiasm.

A couple of weeks after we'd learned I was ovulating, which was a reassuring thing to know, we decided to put in a vegetable garden. Raised beds, the whole bit. We picked up some soil from a garden centre. It looked dead. I doubted it would grow anything. I grew up on a farm with horses, and we'd always had a great garden, so I did some searching on Craigslist and found someone giving away horse shit at a farm about an hour outside of the city. We packed up the car and headed out to fill our trunk.

On the way back, trunk full of shit, we were talking about the general situation, and I did some math in my head and realized I was late. Just a few days. We debated putting off checking, joking about the high price of pregnancy tests, but when we stopped at a dollar store near our house for a trowel and a bucket for the garden, we picked up a few tests as well.

As Matt unloaded the car, I went upstairs to take it.

I remember taking a couple of tests to confirm and then going down to tell him, a little in shock, that it was positive. I remember my heart swelling. I remember us taking another one. I remember our hearts collectively swelling a little more.

We confirmed our pregnancy a couple of days later in the office of our family doctor, who was more than happy to say he'd told us to relax and it would happen and all the well-meaning but asinine things people say to people who struggle with infertility. It felt okay to hear them, to laugh about them a little.

I started spotting at about seven weeks. My doctor said he was still cautiously optimistic and sent me for an ultrasound. I saw the heartbeat, impossibly small but somehow vibrant and full all the same.

I kept bleeding. In my gut, I knew my pregnancy was done. An ultrasound, with an insensitive technician in an ultrasound clinic with stains on the carpet that I will never visit again, confirmed it to be true.

Knowing it was done and being done were two very different things. I miscarried for around a month, through a week of waiting for it to happen on its own and a failed round of misoprostol, which stopped the bleeding for a few days but didn't finish the job. I was in and out of work and forever grateful for a boss who gave me permission to leave as needed. I left at lunchtime a lot that month. It was like reliving a nightmare every single day.

Finally, after two weeks of post-pregnancy bleeding on and off and seeing several of my doctor's colleagues while he was on vacation, who were reluctant to book me for a dilation and curettage (D&C), I landed back in my doctor's office. He took one look at shattered me, pulled in a few favours, and found me a clinic on the other side of town for a D&C the next day.

This clinic was full of people who were mostly not in our situation, but despite that, I had a moment where I was grateful we live in a country where all women get to make this choice and had access to the service I was utilizing. We all shared a desperation of sorts, after all, for a life we felt was the right one for us, even though our circumstances differed. I left Matt in the waiting room and filled out some paperwork in a small office. Here I found out I'd missed my RhoGAM shot, so it was administered by a tiny nurse who was somewhat in shock that, given the number of medical people I'd seen, it had been missed on my chart. (If you're reading this and you have a negative blood type and your partner doesn't, and you're planning to conceive, you should ask your doctor about this or look it up.)

For the rest of my medicalized life, there will be a line on my permanent file that reads that I had an abortion on May 23, 2013. I don't remember it. I remember waking up and lying on a chaise in a room with a bunch of other women. I remember eating an oatmeal cookie and drinking some juice. I remember vomiting on our front lawn when we returned home.

The bleeding slowed down and stopped after that. The crying did not.

They tell you lots of things after you miscarry. They tell you that now you know you can get pregnant, and you're supposed to be happy about that. They tell you that you're extra fertile for the few months after a loss. They tell you this, then in the next breath tell you that you can resume trying with your next cycle, but you shouldn't try until you're ready. But that you're extra fertile and it's a short window. But that you should wait until you're ready.

It's circular, exhausting nonsense.

We'd booked a trip to Italy before we found out we were pregnant, and when we'd found out we were pregnant, we'd joked about my skipping out on wine and resting a lot. I imagined getting winded climbing Cinque Terre and touring the Colosseum out of breath. I'd bought some new duds that were early-bump friendly. I got my period on the plane. It was a horrific bloodbath that lasted a few days and was unlike anything I'd ever experienced. I somehow ended up in a seat by the bathroom on our red-eye flight, which was good, but also horrible because it meant my seat got bumped by other passengers every time I finally fell asleep.

The trip was a good distraction. I got so drunk that I threw up a couple of times. Those who know me know that this is very out of character. We had sex a lot. Not in a romantic-sex-in-Italy-way, but in a void-filling, frantically-needing-optimism way. We longingly joked that it would be a good story, getting pregnant in Italy. It would be the kind of thing we'd embarrass our hypothetical kid with in the future.

We didn't get pregnant.

The next month, my period was late. We stocked up on dollar-store pregnancy tests. We weren't pregnant. I kept crying, often late into the night. Matt suggested that maybe I should talk to someone. I furiously refused. I should have talked to someone, though.

We both should have.

I know other people who have seemingly moved on quickly after a loss. I feel like any feelings on the subject are as valid as a woman's right to choose. If I think back on why I was so upset day in and day out, it was because part of me felt like we'd missed our only chance and that my loss would come to define us. That it was rare and amazing that it had happened at all. It was 10 years of anxiety realized. The worst-case scenario playing out.

I blamed myself. I'd had some wine before I'd known. I'd carried heavy soil for the garden. I'd wished it had happened after we'd gone to Italy. Or in Italy.

In hindsight, this is all utter bullshit. It was very real at the time, however.

I didn't want to be around anyone who was pregnant. I didn't want to be with kids. I left several events and several public spaces because I found seeing babies in carriers, kids in strollers, all of it incredibly overwhelming. I unfollowed my closest friends on social media. I felt like I couldn't breathe. I took my temperature every morning, but the graphs were nonsensical, and I felt like I failed every time I got up to pee around five in the morning and messed up my charting. The pressure consumed me.

My period was late in December. Like two weeks late. I wonder now if this was a missed miscarriage because it was a stuff-of-nightmares period. I didn't take a test. I sort of wish I had, but I just couldn't. I stood in front of the pregnancy tests at the drug store, our dollar-store stash optimistically diminished, and blinked at them, unwilling to face either outcome, as though I was in fertility purgatory.

Our due date would have been Christmas Eve. I spent this day in Florida fighting with my parents in their tiny house because they really didn't acknowledge my pain and just kept suggesting I have a drink or find a way to be optimistic.

Again, I should have seen someone.

A close colleague, who knew my situation, insensitively sent out a pregnancy announcement with three pairs of hiking boots, one impossibly tiny set wedged in the middle of two, with some line about adding a new adventurer to their group. She included me, along with a very long list of people. I cried at my desk.

The next day, Ariel, my co-editor on this project, enthusiastically told me she was expecting. I was very nonplussed about it and felt awful for being cold and distant with her.

I didn't like who I was becoming.

In January, we went to see my doctor again, and after I broke down crying, he agreed to refer us to a fertility clinic but advised us that it might take a while.

The clinic called a week later with a cancellation appointment. I presumed this meant someone had gotten pregnant. I hated them, just a little.

Going to the fertility clinic gave me something I'd desperately needed: validation.

We weren't being impatient. It wasn't a case of just relaxing and waiting for it to happen. I had PCOS. I had a blocked tube that needed unblocking. An appointment was scheduled to have that procedure done. Cycle monitoring indicated I hadn't ovulated that month because my hormones were out of whack. Matt and I both felt better. Proactive. Like we were moving in some sort of direction instead of hopelessly spiralling or screaming into a canyon with weathered and faded "just relax" stickers coating the walls. I felt resigned to a medicalized path, and that felt okay. Our doctor was kind and empathetic.

In February, I started another round of cycle monitoring and was written a prescription for Clomid that I was due to start taking with my cycle in March. I went out and picked up ovulation predictor kits from a dollar store as a last-ditch attempt. They lit up midcycle, right on time. On Valentine's Day, we went out and got corresponding tattoos, huge *Moonrise Kingdom*–themed ones, on our sides. It was awful and painful. Bloody and swollen, we awkwardly did it that night, careful to avoid the bandages, laughing the whole time.

Sometime around then, out of my nonblocked left tube, the egg that would become my kid was kicked out. We found out mid-March we were expecting. The doctor said it probably had something to do with the hysterosalpingogram, which can also increase your fertility the cycle after you have it. We'd been told that, but I'd ignored it at the time, not wanting to get too caught up in false optimism.

Because we were at a fertility clinic, we spent the first 14 weeks of our pregnancy monitored to the hilt. Weekly ultrasounds. Blood tests. Techs who showed us everything and reassured us constantly. It was first-degree coddling and an experience that is unlike what so many women experience after a loss. It was exactly what we needed to survive the first trimester.

I had imagined that once we conceived and had passed the first trimester, my infertility concerns and the trauma of a decade of living with them would dissolve into thin air. I imagined the crater my miscarriage had left was perfectly baby-sized. I'm not sure what I thought would happen. Neither Matt or I felt much throughout our pregnancy except for an impending sense of doom, and it wasn't until we heard our son cry that anything felt like it was going to be okay.

The thing that people don't tell you about infertility is that it exists within the mind alongside the physical symptoms. A lot of it is in your head. I don't say this in a "just relax" context. I mean your condition becomes part of who you are, how you define yourself. It's not necessarily a negative; struggling to get pregnant has made me a much more empathetic person. It's made me more considerate of others. It's taught me not to ask about things that people ask when they're making small talk that cuts to the core of a person's psyche. It's taught me to never make assumptions about people's choices.

It's made me a better listener; someone who doesn't shy away from hard conversations. I'm now someone who easily volunteers to go to the grave of a baby that another mother in this volume was having a hard time visiting for the first time. It's why, since my miscarriage, I've been on the other side of dozens of conversations with women who need someone to throw them a life preserver in dark times. I haven't told them that everything will be okay, but that they will be fine and will make and know their own version of okay. That they will find purpose, not meaning, in their situation. Because they are stronger than they know.

The flip side is that it has left me darker. In a way, it's logical; a death within your body is bound to have an emotional impact far beyond the medical process of ending a pregnancy. It's made me less sure about many things that seem like they should be givens. It's also taken me to the depths of my personal determination and my ability to endure. I can say, with unwavering certainty, that I would have done anything to be a mother. The how became less important, over time.

14

THE PIECES OF
ME AND YOU

Neusa Arraial

SINCE MY TEENAGE YEARS, I had been convinced that I did not want to be a mom. Nothing about motherhood spoke or appealed to me. I was so sure of this that on the very first date with my husband, I told him I did not want to have children. He did, but he loved and married me anyway.

For 12 years of marriage, Hugo quietly and patiently chipped away at the cement wall that I had built to keep motherhood out of my life. By January 2015, he had finally made enough of a crack, and I agreed to hold his hand to fearfully jump into parenting — on one condition: I was going to give it a shot for three months only. If we didn't conceive within three months, I was done. My family doctor laughed when I told her this, but three months later, there I was in her office, looking for the official confirmation that I was, in fact, pregnant.

Physically, the first month of my pregnancy was awesome. No morning sickness, no nausea, no food aversions — it was as if I weren't even pregnant. Mentally, though, the first month of my pregnancy was a battlefield filled with fear and self-doubt. I was determined to keep my life as it always had been and would not give in to using my pregnancy as an excuse for anything — especially changing out of high heels into flats. I had spent years establishing standards for myself that I was prepared to fight for, regardless of what or who entered my life.

At around the 10-week mark, I started spotting. What followed for the next 11 weeks was increased bleeding, frequent visits to the hospital emergency room, two weeks of bedrest including one week of hospitalization, a hemoglobin blood level of 70 (normal is from 120 to 140), which almost led to a blood transfusion, and finally a diagnosis of a detached placenta. I was immediately placed on the list for an appointment at Mount Sinai Hospital in Toronto for a second opinion and additional monitoring. Unfortunately for me, that meant a two-week waiting period.

On the hot evening of August 31, 2015, I did not feel right. I started cramping, and although at first I refused to make yet another trip to the emergency room, I listened to my husband and together we drove to the hospital. Because I was 21 weeks into my pregnancy, well into my second trimester, the nurses in the emergency room sent me to the labour and delivery unit. After an initial examination by the obstetrician on call, my husband and I were told that our baby was on its way. At 21 weeks, my cervix was already fully dilated, and transferring me to Mount Sinai Hospital would put me at risk of delivering my baby en route.

The nurse on duty found Jude's heartbeat before prepping me for labour. That was the last time I heard my baby's heart, before my body failed me.

On September 1, 2015, at 2:19 a.m., Hugo and I met Jude face to face. Our sweet baby boy was born already sleeping. He was 1.04 pounds and 11 inches long. A tiny perfect little boy who in a second showed us what it's truly like to love unconditionally. We were both in shock. From the time we had driven to the hospital at 10:30 p.m. to the time I delivered Jude, the events and conversations that took place sent us into autopilot. We had no time to think or process the reality that now hit us like a freight train. What we thought was going to be a routine visit to the hospital ended up being the end of our lives as we knew them.

After we were released from the hospital and said goodbye to Jude, a thoughtful nurse took a picture of him. As a part-time photographer, I've captured moments of pure love: from weddings to family portraits to newborn photos. And yet the thought of capturing a photo of my own sweet little boy never crossed my traumatized mind.

Fifteen months later I found myself staring at a composed framed image I had become all too familiar with. The stark contrast between the white and the black, complemented by varying shades of grey, surrounding the formation of human lips. The tiny perfect saliva bubble captured at the right second when the shutter of the camera was released. As I carefully examined the photo, I barely noticed the technical brilliance of it. All I could focus on was the image of what had become unattainable subject matter. As I had so many times in the months leading up to that moment, I wondered, *How did I get here?*

After losing Jude, the idea of trying for another pregnancy was a pressure-cooker topic for my husband and me, filled with many conflicting emotions and fears. We were often triggered by unhelpful advice or comments or the presence of pregnant women during our roller-coaster ride of grief. Not only was I robbed of a lifetime with my son, I was robbed of the ignorantly blissful experience of pregnancy. Once you enter the child-loss community, you become strikingly aware of all the possible things that can lead to the death of your unborn child. No percentage or odds configuration brings reassurance to a subsequent pregnancy once you've become part of a child-loss statistic.

The thought of experiencing yet another loss was frightening, but it wasn't what I actually feared the most. In a way, I had figured out how to cope with the grief and found ways to manage it. What terrified me was the thought of having a healthy pregnancy and child only to then resent it. "What if we end up with a lemon?" I kept asking my husband. The thought of ending up with a child who was not like Jude, who we had immortalized as perfect, was terrifying. I struggled with guilt surrounding the fact that another child would get a chance at life but Jude hadn't. *Why not Jude?*

With all that in mind, during our fourth month of grieving, we decided to face our fears and conceded to the idea of another pregnancy. Confident in our ability to conceive, I once again set my expectations for a short timeline, bracing for the anxiety-filled nine-month waiting period that I would be faced with.

But after 12 months of trying to conceive with no success, my husband and I agreed to go to a fertility clinic to ensure that there was nothing medically out of the ordinary with either of us. I had firmly planted the stake in the ground: I would never be one of those women obsessed with the idea of getting pregnant. I would not take temperatures, track days on a calendar, or pee on ovulation sticks, waiting for a flashing happy face to tell me when to engage in intercourse with my husband. Yet there I was, signing up for just that.

I had once been childless by choice. Going back to that status was no longer an option. My reality was that I had a child. I was a mother. The difference was that my motherhood didn't extend beyond the borders of my heart. And even though I had found ways to mother my son without him being physically present, I still had an overflowing reserve of love to give to someone. Someone I could physically hold. Physically love. Physically mother.

In the first 12 months that followed the loss of Jude, I'd been able to contain the overflow of that love, tending to it with the hope that another child would soon be present in our lives. But when another child didn't come, the overflow drowned the hope.

In the 10 months that followed our first visit to the fertility clinic, I was probed, pricked, and examined countless times. I became the ringmaster of multitasking and emotional disguise, juggling work meetings and fertility clinic appointments, often starting my day at 5:30 a.m. in order to race to the clinic for their first appointment slot at 7:00, all the while still grieving my son.

I continued balancing work and fertility appointments as I watched my relationship with my husband weaken. Both of us were losing sight of why we were even participating in this circus at all. *What was the end goal again?* In the midst of grieving the absence of our son, Jude; the loss of our perfectly planned life together; and the loss of our core selves, we had forgotten what we were playing for exactly.

In an attempt to comfort us, our fertility doctor assured us that we were not alone. Many clients of hers, young professionals mainly, struggled to conceive, simply because of the combination of stress levels in their professional and personal lives. Eliminating or reducing stress was part of the solution. Alternatives were also presented: adoption, surrogacy, and in vitro fertilization, all great options for those who struggled with conception. But in my mind, those were not options for me. Medically, there was nothing wrong with me. The machine was working perfectly — just not producing anything.

But the fact that there was nothing medically wrong with either my husband or me nearly drove me mad. All around me I saw pregnant women from all walks of life, in so many different situations, who had never struggled to get pregnant, and I couldn't help but feel jealous that there I was, childless after child loss. I couldn't wrap my head around that concept. I couldn't understand why I was simply not able to achieve what I had had before, and what so many others around me managed to have. All I wanted was the opportunity to finish what I had started.

Every woman who has signed up for the infertility clinic circus will tell you that the last two weeks of her cycle are pure and utter torture. The waiting, the hope, the caution of every move are all wrapped up in a time bomb ticking away, waiting for the fateful day when its trigger fuse will be lit. During the 11th month of my infertility treatment, my fuse was lit. Surprisingly, the culprit wasn't my negative pregnancy-test result, the one I had come to expect every month. This time, the culprit was a good friend of mine. A friend who had endured the hardship of infertility herself, who now had a nine-month-old daughter and was announcing, with a simple text, that she had a surprise. Another baby was on the way. That text triggered the bomb inside of me, leaving pieces of hope, grief, anger, jealousy, resentment, and love splattered everywhere.

A few weeks after we had lost Jude, someone planted a seed of an idea that had resonated with me ever since. It was during that cleanup that I remembered the idea, which is that our children choose us. My friend had miraculously been chosen again. Someone had chosen her. She hadn't undergone any treatment. No medical assistance. No stress level management. No control. She was simply chosen. The idea gave me comfort.

My new self grasped on to that perspective and ran with it. Holding it close to my heart, I gracefully acknowledged and bowed down to my status of childless after child loss and decided I was no longer going to be held captive by it. I was no longer going to sit in the cold, stark white medical waiting room of the fertility clinic with my cycle-monitoring charts and my notion that I could control any of it.

So I stopped. I stopped trying to be selected. I stopped banging my head against the wall trying for another pregnancy. Instead, I focused on nurturing and nourishing my childless self that so desperately needed to be tended to.

The reality was that so much of myself was lost in the process of losing Jude. Core pieces of me just disappeared into thin air in a matter of seconds. The pieces that hung by a few threads later lost their grip and vanished like a plastic bag caught in the wind. Very few remained; none remained intact. All that was left were fragmented pieces of the person I used to be, the person I currently was, and the person I had vowed never to be. I was completely out of sync.

A feeling of unfamiliarity, emptiness, and confusion filled the void left by those core pieces that had once stood within me, firmly and confidently rooted. That unfamiliar feeling sprawled into all aspects of my life, almost becoming part of my new core. As my grief journey bent and changed, I became more disturbed by the consistent presence of this unfamiliarity with myself, with who I had become after losing Jude. I knew that I had to change it. In order to know who I was again, I had to take time to get to know the new pieces of me that remained scattered, the ones I had yet to integrate with the few pieces of my old self that remained.

A friend had once suggested to me that I should take up knitting as a resource to help me cope. And so I did. Surprised by my newfound activity, my husband asked me what I was knitting. "I don't know," I answered. That was the liberating truth. I was starting on a journey of rebuilding myself without any preconceived notions of who I wanted to become or where I was going. Just as I had no idea what the end result of my knitting would be, I had no idea what the end result of piecing myself back together would be. I just knew that I had to knit the pieces together. I would fuse the pieces of me that were left behind after losing Jude with the new pieces of me that I found in the rubble of my broken heart. I would start over, bringing together the old and the new.

As the yarn twined between my fingers, shaping itself into something as the days went on, I carefully started knitting pieces of myself together, too. The first piece was my ability to be resourceful. I found myself searching YouTube for step-by-step videos on how to cast on, the very first step to knitting. As I worked my way through the exercise, I noticed the stitches were tighter and closer, and the pattern more pronounced. Those elements were also elements I started to notice within me. Since giving myself permission to wipe the canvas clean and start rebuilding, I, too, was becoming stronger, more self-aware, and more defined in who I was and who I wanted to be. From there I continued to build and continued to learn.

My quest for a subsequent pregnancy after losing Jude had been fuelled by the idea that I simply wanted to finish what I had started. But what I soon realized was that I actually had finished what I had started — it just didn't have the ending that I thought it would. Having another child would not be a continuation — it would just be a new start, a new beginning with its own set of challenges, fears, and joys, experienced by a new version of me. That realization and understanding allowed me to knit in another piece, the piece of me that was accepting of the fact that I may never have another child, that my experience of motherhood might remain physically invisible.

As I learned to feel whole again, I leaned in closer to the idea that our children choose us. Jude chose me. Out of every single woman in the universe, Jude chose *me*. I don't know why he chose me, but I know that he did. The person he chose is very different than the person that I have become after becoming his mom. I look at myself in the mirror and know that the reflection I currently see is a much gentler, kinder, compassionate reflection than the previous one.

Hanging on the inside of my walk-in closet is a five-by-seven-inch chalkboard frame that I use as a gratitude reminder board. In white chalk, I often scribble mantras or identify moments of gratitude to help keep me grounded while healing. After months of being reminded how grateful I am for the ability to travel with my husband, I wiped away the chalk dust and stared at the clean chalkboard.

Picking up the chalk pen, I carefully wrote the words out: "Let them once again choose you."

I shared the perspective with my therapist in a session I had the following week and she approached it with caution. "What if you don't get pregnant again? I'm afraid that may spiral you into the thought process that you aren't good enough to be chosen again," she noted.

I thought about her question, but felt that was not going to be the case. I knew now that this new version of me was much better than the old version of me. And if the old version was chosen by Jude, then the new version would be chosen by someone else. A different soul, looking to be loved by me, too, but differently. I also knew that even if there was nobody else, if I wasn't once again chosen, that the piece of me that had come to accept my childless self was tightly knit into the patchwork of my new core self and that I would be okay.

I knew that because I had knitted it in myself.

15

MISSED CONCEPTIONS

Kelly MacCready

IN SOME WAYS, it was so long ago that I tell myself I don't remember. Yet I know the truth is that, most often, I don't let myself remember.

Infertility is not a place I like to revisit — these are not happy memories. I am shocked, even now, at the lengths I went to in order to have something I was convinced was necessary for my happiness, my fulfillment. My completion. Infertility, for me, spanned almost a decade, and I can't remember if I miscarried six or seven times — I guess it depends which ones I count. And oddly enough, some count more than others, depending on how much hope I had instilled in the growing tissue in my body at the time. It seems to me now that I had no control but was desperate for some. And I still don't know or understand (nor do the doctors) how my body worked and did what it did: how it decided which babies to discard and which babies to keep. There is one particular conception, one loss, I still think about with regard to the person she might be today. I picture her with her red hair flowing in the wind and wonder if she would be different. Of course she would be.

My infertility experience, in all honesty, is one of the stories that drove me most crazy while I was trying to "complete" my family, because of how society interprets its message and re-creates it, sending it out to countless women trying to create their own families. I do this all the time. I analyze, interpret, reflect, and give my opinions before even telling the story. And the whole purpose of this is to share my story. So here it is.

Our first son was conceived in July 2000 in northern Ontario beside a gorgeous quiet lake. I was 31 and, truth be told, he was the product of the first unprotected sex I had ever had. I thought I was capital-F Fertile. But motherhood was a more intense and all-encompassing experience than I could have imagined, so I didn't rush to have a second child. In fact, I have a vague memory of being unsure whether I wanted another child. In reality, I was relishing and enjoying my first child and was not ready to share myself or him. Part of me still blames myself for waiting and wonders what might have happened if I hadn't.

I was 35 when we started trying for a second child. It was great fun for a while, until I began wasting money on home pregnancy tests. It's just so tricky when the symptoms of pregnancy — sore breasts, slight cramping, food cravings — can actually be caused by your period coming. I grew to hate those tiny sticks. They had so much power with their little lines that seemed to come and go indiscriminately. It took at least a year to get a positive on one of them, and then I quickly grew to distrust the tests because twice they told me yes and then the blood started and the cramps worsened and the hCG hormone levels at the doctor's office plummeted.

Those were my early miscarriages. When I talked to anyone about them, I was told it was common and nothing to stress about, and I already had a child, so I would surely have another soon. My doctor attributed these "little losses" (her words) to my age and told me not to worry. I was obviously fertile since I was "conceiving something."

Another year and a half and 12 boxes of First Response later, I knew it was a strong pregnancy when the little lines on the pregnancy sticks got darker and darker every day and the hCG level was in the tens of thousands by the time I got to the doctor's office. Me, my partner, and my son were all so excited for that pregnancy, having tried for so many years to conceive. In fact, it felt like a whole community was excited; I was immersed in a group of families with two children each and thought I might join their ranks. But at 13.5 weeks, I started to bleed copiously and cramp horribly. This miscarriage was in some ways the worst one. It was the most physically painful and long lasting, the one that caught me by surprise (I made it to the second trimester!), and the one during which, when I returned from the ultrasound to check for a heartbeat, my five-and-a-half-year-old asked me, "Where's the baby? Did you leave it at the hospital? When can we go get it?"

The awful pain and the passing of large masses through me and the endless blood and the passing out and the eventual emergency dilation and curettage (D&C) at four o'clock in the morning were almost cathartic. I let myself cry and sob for that loss. I was just coming out of anaesthesia when a kindly doctor touched my arm and said, "It was good that we went in there, Kelly. There was still a lot of tissue to be cleared out, and if it makes you feel any better, the baby died a few weeks ago. But you'll be able to try again once your body recovers."

I took so much from those kind words in the middle of the night. I would not let my body surprise me again. I would know everything about subsequent pregnancies. I would not go around thinking I was pregnant when I wasn't, only to be crushed. I wanted to take control.

In some ways, my real journey of infertility, or fertility treatment, began here. By that time, my experiences trying to conceive my second child had warranted referral to a fertility clinic. In 2007, I entered the world of cycle monitoring, intrauterine insemination (IUI), and in vitro fertilization (IVF). I thought this might give me some control.

Anyone who has undergone cycle monitoring is familiar with the ups and downs of closely following your own reproductive cycle with technical assistance, technicians, and assistants. I imagine each one of us approaches it differently, but who could not be affected by administering needles to themselves in the hopes of growing more eggs, watching their own eggs grow and mature on a monitor, watching their own lining thicken, and seeing all the roadblocks in their own body that stand in the way of conceiving that desired child? In my case, the roadblocks were polyps, cysts, and fibroids, but I was assured by my specialist these were not insurmountable.

I spent two more years doing IUI without ever conceiving. My specialist consistently said that she was shocked and she had a very hopeful feeling every time we did another round of insemination. In some ways, those years are now a blur to me. A blur of early morning lineups with other women who were having their cycles assessed and inspected. What I remember most vividly is how I surprised myself with my ability to give myself the needles and find patches of unbruised skin ready for puncture. My partner couldn't even look. And how much it hurt physically to ovulate multiple eggs at a time and how much it hurt emotionally to have the nurse call with the negative hCG result, especially because I had already spent the money and peed on a stick. I knew I wasn't pregnant.

Those two years ended with a ruptured cyst on an ovary that led me to surgery, where they discovered I was "riddled with endometriosis." I was diagnosed with secondary infertility and my doctor said she didn't think I could conceive without IVF. I was so tired of trying to get pregnant then and disappointed in my own inability to conceive. I didn't want IVF and it cost so much money, since none of it was covered at the time. My partner and I decided to take a break and pursue adoption, which we had also been considering for years.

At the end of 2010, I returned to my fertility clinic and doctor, ready to try IVF, ready to try anything. I was almost 42 and the test they conducted showed low ovarian reserve, so my doctor cautioned me that I would not have a good chance of conceiving with my eggs. She told me that the best approach would be with donor eggs and that she thought I had a 90 percent chance of getting pregnant with a donor and my partner's sperm. This sounded like music to my ears and the answer to my years-long longing for another child. I dreamed of the child that I would carry and nurse, but hold no biological relation to, and somehow got a certain thrill from the beauty of the different ways to create and conceive families. I pored over donor profiles and felt an urgency to get things moving as quickly as possible — perhaps this was my age or the growing gap in years that would exist between my children. In retrospect, all I can remember is a sense of desperation in moving this process along. A part of me wishes I could contact all the people involved in that process and apologize for what I assume were interactions that, on my part, were filled with stress, tension, desperation, and a desire for control. I think I was rude to some people and I'm sorry now. I also remember believing deeply that I would have a child conceived through these donor eggs.

My belief in my second child was profound. I thought for sure this was the way she would come to us. I remember the day we found out that 12 embryos of varying grades had grown from the donor eggs and sperm. We were so hopeful and felt we were sure to conceive. I mean, with 12 eggs, I was imagining having our baby and afterward donating the extra embryos to other people who wanted children. After all, I would be 43 when I gave birth, so I might not feel I was able to have another. Each embryo transfer went "wonderfully," according to the technicians, and in total resulted in five pregnancies, though ultimately each ended in a loss. The first one, the one that resulted in a positive pregnancy test, attached a little too early along the way — in my Fallopian tube.

I remember the beginning of that pregnancy as euphoric. It had worked! Donor eggs had worked and I conceived with a doubling hCG right away, just as the doctor had said I would. I was feeling fantastic at six weeks and my blood work was good, so the ultrasound to check on the pregnancy was routine. I remember the atmosphere in the room turned fetid when the technician couldn't find the fetus and called someone else in to look. And then they called someone else and then someone else. And finally my doctor came, and her worried eyes strained at the monitor while the ultrasound wand probed around to places it had not probed before, higher and more difficult to reach. My body was producing convincing amounts of hCG but no heartbeat could be found anywhere.

My doctor was genuinely sad for me when she told me it was probably ectopic and I needed to take methotrexate to ensure it didn't keep growing. She patted me many times and told me she felt very sure that, since I had conceived this one and I had so many embryos left, I would soon be a mother again. This was just a little blip along the way. My feelings of desperation grew along with anger at my body for failing me again in a new and different way, but I didn't give up hope. I bled out that conception and waited to be ready for another embryo transfer. I had nine left. I still had many chances.

The truth is I confuse the last three miscarriages. They tumble over each other and I lose track of the bleeding and the thickening of my lining and the hCG levels doubling and even tripling and the appointments where there were heartbeats and the appointments where there were none. A part of me knew I should slow down and wait a little longer between embryo transfers. When I look back on that period, I remember I took a bereavement leave from work but I can't remember after which miscarriage.

One of them held such hope, such promise. I was pregnant and my hCG levels were doubling. This time we were careful and so we monitored the pregnancy even more closely with additional ultrasounds. Each time the heartbeat was there, clear and strong, but I was nervous and anxious because I had had so many losses. Everything was fine, my doctor kept assuring me. And so I dreamed of the second child and imagined her and hoped. And then the bleeding started — it always did, eventually. I went back to the doctor, and miraculously — and this is why I remember it — the baby was still there. Sure I was bleeding; it had happened, and yes, it happened in some pregnancies where women still carried to full term. So I went back home bleeding but knowing there was still a beating heart in there and that plenty of women bleed but still carry the baby.

The blood kept coming and increased and clotted and was relentless. It was Easter weekend and my doctor wasn't there, nor was she on call, so the nurse recommended waiting. So I waited, bleeding, hopeful, and desperate. I found out on Tuesday that there was no more heartbeat. My son was almost 11 now and he no longer asked innocent questions about where the baby went. He was stoic and comforting. I remember him saying, "You can put your head on my shoulder if you want, Mom." But I felt guilty, like I should be comforting him.

I remember the last miscarriage vividly. It was the last chance, the last hope. Actually, I'm not sure if I really had any hope left. I mean, my uterus had already killed nine embryos by then. That's how it felt. I remember feeling incredibly hormonal. To be fair, I was taking a lot of hormones to prepare me for the transfer and I was an emotional wreck. *Wreck* being the operative word, because it was exactly how my body felt. But I got a positive hCG on that last pregnancy. I remember the fleeting hope. I remember talking to myself, saying, *Okay, you're pregnant. But don't get your hopes up. You are pregnant. But you have a long way to go. Take it easy. Go slow.* And I remember the phone call that said that my hCG levels were not doubling. They were dropping. I would miscarry. I would miscarry again.

I was so tired of miscarrying. I was so tired of the emotional ups and downs of all of it. I remember giving up. I remember losing all hope and deciding never to contact the clinic again. I was supposed to come in for a follow-up, but I could never get myself to dial the number again and I ached every time I passed the clinic. I went camping the weekend I found out I would have my final miscarriage. I figured, *What the hell?* I was going to miscarry anyway; it might as well be while I was camping. I remember when the bleeding started and being held up by two friends in the shower and the tissue coming out of my body and crying and crying and crying. I don't go back to that memory often. And I have never revisited it with those friends.

And then there is the epilogue to my infertility story. The epilogue changes everything. It changes my memories and changes the way it is shared and heard and read and felt. It may change your reading of this story, too.

EPILOGUE

My first child was always a salve to the wound of missed conceptions and miscarriages. I always knew I should feel grateful, and I did and do feel so grateful for him, but I also felt I had less right to be disappointed or pained by my losses because I already had one child. But pain doesn't work that way — it just existed and seemed to be only compounded by guilt and shame when I berated myself for wanting more children. There was a reckoning that happened in the wake of my last miscarriage, an evaluation or a settlement in my life. I remember talking to myself again: *Okay, so you won't have another child, but you already have a beautiful and wonderful child. You are already so lucky. You have tried and you're almost 43 and it's time you accept the situation.* In the fall of 2011, after my final miscarriage, I began to accept that we were a beautiful family of three and we would stay that way. And I did feel grateful.

Another two years went by. I turned 44 and we were enjoying a wonderful summer. We were blessed with time by a beautiful lake. Not a quiet lake this time, like with my son. This time it was a strong and fierce one in southern Ontario. Many weeks later my period was very late, my breasts were sore, and I had cramping. But this meant nothing to me. This was life. Periods are weird and menopause was on its way. I let more weeks pass, until the day my 7:00 a.m. shift started with a coffee that made me throw up. Coffee never did that to me ... unless I was pregnant. I ran to the drugstore and bought one of those sticks I thought I was all done with.

The line lit up in a millisecond. I remember the shock and disbelief. I called my old fertility doctor, who was equally shocked and asked me to come in right away. An ultrasound probe confirmed a growing egg sac. I remember the fear, the caution, and the anxiety I carried with me for the next nine months. So many people asked if I was excited and to that I always thought, *I'm not excited to have another miscarriage.* I simultaneously felt guilty for thinking so negatively.

It was an anxious pregnancy — but it was full term. I turned 45 and weeks later gave birth to my daughter. She is 13 years younger than her brother and a biological production of the same two people that produced him. She's not who I thought she'd be and I'm forever grateful for her: for her coming to this world and for who she is. She is the epilogue to infertility and she truly isn't what I expected. Yet I'm keenly aware that she softens the blows of infertility that I bore. All those years I spent trying to have a second child were full of advice to "relax, let go and it'll happen." Oh, how I tried to do that. But I never could. Looking back, I realize that even when we stopped our fertility treatment, I never let go and I never really gave up.

People have asked me, but the truth is I have absolutely no advice for anyone going through infertility. I have only my stories and the knowledge of how much loss can hurt. And how much love can heal.

16
NOT A SPRINT

Lauren Simmons

THERE'S THIS SAYING: It's a marathon, not a sprint. I hear this said often in modern parlance: before the holiday party season, an intense period of work, a gruelling conference, or a family vacation. The idea, I think, is to remind oneself that the period ahead requires endurance, fortitude, pacing, and soundness of mind and body. It's no surprise, then, that I considered this my mantra when I was undergoing fertility treatment.

It's ironic, really, that I frame my infertility experience with a running metaphor, since one of the first things the fertility doctor told me, on the day I started treatment, was that I'd have to stop running if I wanted to get pregnant. It was not a surprise to me; I understood that my usual activity level of biking to work a few days a week, running a few days a week, and going to the gym most days would be a focus of attention, and perhaps even a cause for concern, as I began the treatment process. Nonetheless, I was struck by the finiteness of the doctor's statement. Like so much else she said that day, there was no flexibility, no nuance in her approach: You can't run, but you can lift weights. Don't drink more than three drinks in a night, but one drink is okay. Oh, and don't forget to keep your stress levels low. A fine thing to tell someone you've also just told to stop running. There was no way I could process everything that was happening, no way I could reduce my stress, like everyone said I needed to, *without* running.

Running is, in some ways, my oldest relationship. I wasn't an athletic kid. My extracurricular time at school was spent in choir rehearsals or backstage at musicals. But once I moved out on my own, in my second year of university, going to the gym a few times a week became one of the ways I got out of the house, giving me a routine to centre my days and weeks around in the dark of Montreal winter. I started running when I moved back to Toronto for the summer that year, again, as a way to get out of the house. Though in summer it was more about getting space for myself, away from my family. Running stayed with me throughout the tumult of my university years, graduating, and moving back to Toronto to begin my career. Running was a constant companion I could return to for peace, calm, and quiet. My dedication to exercise, to moving my body in functional ways, was a part of my identity when I met my husband, and it stayed central to who I was throughout my 30s. At various times, I was more enamoured with one sport than another — I spent one winter obsessed with BodyAttack classes, another spring with spinning and cycling, completing the 200-kilometre Ride to Conquer Cancer in 2008 and 2010 — but I always came back to running. Putting on a pair of shoes is the easiest way for me to get back to myself, and while I knew I had to moderate my passion in order to get pregnant, I didn't respond well to this new reality.

We knew we wanted to be parents. I knew I wanted to co-parent with my partner. So a few years after we got married, I went off the pill, which I'd been on for over a decade. After a few months, I discovered I didn't have a regular period, which caused my doctor to refer us to a fertility clinic. This was an accelerated process; we didn't have the months or years of trying on our own before our referral. This meant that we were pretty unfamiliar with the frustration and disappointment inherent in fertility treatment. As a perfectionist, I was particularly unprepared for how disheartening it can be to do all the right things but not get the desired results.

When you're training for a marathon, everything in your life has to support your training in some way or another. You need to eat foods that will adequately fuel your training. You need to rest to recover from training. You need to make adjustments in your workload, volunteer commitments, and social life in order to make room for training. Your loved ones need to understand that you're undergoing something big and need to support you. So the comparisons between fertility treatment and marathon running are apt. But the difference is that when you're training for a marathon, barring injury, your body responds to training. As you put in the miles, the early mornings or late nights, your body adapts; you get faster, able to run longer. With fertility treatment, no matter how much room you make in your life, no matter how many changes you make, your body may not respond. Mine didn't.

I resented fertility treatment from the moment I started it. I resented being told that running, this thing I loved and considered central to my identity, could be holding me back from my dreams of being pregnant. I resented the early mornings at the clinic, elbowing other prospective mothers for first place on the sign-up clipboards for the various procedures. I resented daily blood tests and internal ultrasounds. I resented them for how drained and violated they left me feeling, every day. I resented getting on the subway after all of that and going to work, expected to carry on with my day with no space for me to recover from the ongoing process. I resented that it was clearly my body that was failing as we continued to be unsuccessful in our attempts. I resented the terse and glib nature of some of the professionals at our clinic. I resented having to move through the world with very few of my friends knowing what we were going through, with little to no support or community.

Eventually, after one chemical pregnancy and a whole lot of other failures, after less than half a year of trying (incidentally, about the length of a typical marathon training cycle), I hated fertility treatment so much that I quit. Most runners won't quit training once they've started, unless they get injured or their lives change dramatically in some other way. But I felt strongly that fertility treatment was asking too much of me and taking too much away from me, and I decided that it was not going to work. We stopped going for cycle monitoring, I stopped taking the drugs, and my husband and I went back to being life DINKs (double income, no kids). We didn't talk much about our feelings during this time.

I knew I wanted to try again, eventually, but I wasn't going to be able to do it while working and volunteering and exercising and just generally rushing through life the way I tend to do. I picked a date and told myself that if we weren't pregnant by then, I'd take a leave of absence from work and go back to fertility treatment, ready to make all the necessary sacrifices.

It seemed like the only viable option — I couldn't make space for fertility treatment without first making space for myself to process it, physically and emotionally. My partner supported this proposition, I think particularly because I hadn't closed the door on fertility treatment completely. It was a challenging time for us in many ways. Scores of our friends and acquaintances got pregnant and had kids. We travelled, bought expensive wine, and travelled more. I ran.

In the year that followed my decision to quit fertility treatment, I ramped up my running in a serious way. I trained for my first 30-kilometre race and several half-marathons. After a summer spent running some of my highest mileage, and after a month when I'd run two races in a week, I got pregnant. It was clear to me then that everything about fertility treatment had been wrong for me, from the get-go, and my resentment had been warranted. I was, of course, incredibly lucky that my circumstances had changed and that my body had changed and I was able to get pregnant on my own. We celebrated, told too many too soon, and dreamed big dreams. But as it turns out, my infertility marathon wasn't over. I wasn't even within sight of the finish line.

I lost my first pregnancy. We went in for the 14-week ultrasound, excited to see images, hear a heartbeat, and get a tangible sense that it was all really happening, only to find none of that was true. I was scheduled for a dilation and curettage (D&C) right before the holiday season and spent most of December and January untelling everyone the news and trying to dampen the pain by whatever means necessary. We travelled. I drank. I exercised. I couldn't run, because somehow in the course of the D&C procedure, I strained a muscle in my inner thigh. It was the hardest time in my life, and I couldn't do the one thing I needed to do to process it. And then in March, just as I was healthy and getting back to running, I found out I was pregnant again.

The pregnancy I had after infertility was a gift, the kind of gift you're so excited about that you rip the package open and discard the hand-painted, carefully selected wrapping paper on the floor. The pregnancy I had after my miscarriage was a gift, too, but the kind that you're so grateful for that you almost don't even want to open it — you cherish every part of it, from the ribbon to the last piece of wrapping paper that you carefully fold, storing it for later. My second pregnancy came just before spring, as the world was melting and the temperatures rose and the green returned to the world. I kept running, confident that it was best for my body, and for the baby I was running with. I trained for a half-marathon and ran it at five months, on the same weekend my first baby would have been due.

I'm sure many people have said that pregnancy is a marathon, not a sprint. The nine months spent sharing your body with another being certainly require endurance and keeping an eye on the prize. I was extremely lucky, in that — apart from muscle strains, migraines, scent sensitivity, and nosebleeds — pregnancy agreed with my body. I enjoyed staying active and fuelling my growing baby, equipping my body for the real finish line of labour, which as it turns out, is a different kind of marathon. I was remarkably and uncharacteristically laid back about my pregnancy and preparation for labour. I was prepared to welcome my baby to the world however they wanted to arrive. I wasn't hung up on an unmedicated birth, though I wanted to try. I was ready and willing to accept any outcome that led to a healthy baby, and I wasn't stressed about a birth plan or ideal circumstances for my labour and delivery. Not to begrudge women for whom these things are important, of course — we all process and prepare for this monumental life occasion in the way that works best for us. But for me, after having experienced the marathon of fertility treatment and miscarriage that I did, I was just happy to be at the starting line of this next race. Like every time I line up to run, I had a goal in mind (runners call this the A goal), but I also had subgoals (the B goal, C goal, etc.), and I was willing to accept whatever my body had in it that day.

I had what I understand to be a very typical labour experience. I made it 41 weeks with no sign of action. I started experiencing contractions that were very manageable, so I walked to Starbucks and then later we ordered Thai food. At bedtime, I realized the contractions were getting worse and closer together and I wasn't going to be able to sleep at home, so we headed for the hospital. Despite my self-perception as someone with a high pain tolerance, particularly as a runner, I knew that if I wanted to rest and be my best for the physical task ahead, I wanted pain medication. So I got an epidural and experienced no guilt or remorse. I had contractions overnight, got some medication to speed them along, and gave birth just before noon, about 12 hours after we had checked in. The only qualm I had with my labour was that I was terribly hungry when I entered the pushing phase, having had no solid food since I got the epidural. In hindsight, I should have brought some sports nutrition gels with me. If I ever labour again, I'm definitely going to work on my fuelling (an area where many runners falter as well).

Two years after my daughter's birth, I ran the Chicago Marathon. Two weeks before that marathon, I rolled my ankle, dashing my hopes of achieving a good time in my marathon debut. It was a fluke accident, a misstep off a curb, and it meant that my months of training were all for naught. I spent the next two weeks maxing out my chiropractic and physio benefits, getting acupuncture and soft tissue work and everything else I could throw at the injury, in the hopes that I would be able to line up on race day. I never really mentally prepared for the possibility of not running, just as I had never really envisioned a childless life before my infertility journey began. Had I not been able to run that day, I'm not sure how I would have coped. As it turned out, the disappointment I felt at not being able to run full out for 42.2 kilometres was damped by the euphoria of running my first marathon in a city I love and finishing the whole dang thing while injured.

I had often heard it said, and knew from my experiences running other races, that your mind does strange things when you're running a marathon. You have a lot of time out there on the road to spend with your own self, and you can't control where your mind will go. Much like in meditation or mindfulness, when a thought comes into your head, you can see it, acknowledge it, then send it on its way. When I was running Chicago, my thoughts returned again and again to the baby I lost in my miscarriage. Because I became pregnant again so soon afterward, I never took the time to mourn or acknowledge that loss in any meaningful way. So as I put one foot in front of the other running that race, I took a moment, or several moments, to dedicate my race to that baby. I'll never know why my mind went there that day, but it did.

The marathon was the physical culmination of months of work, yes, months of adjusting my life and making room for the training and recovery. But it was also the result of the mental fortitude it took to get through those months, and through the race itself. Infertility and miscarriage had prepared me for the marathon because they taught me both to trust my body and to ignore my body completely, which one eventually needs to do in a marathon, as well as to trust my mind. In the five years that I experienced infertility, miscarriage, pregnancy, childbirth, and being a parent to a newborn, the mental fortitude I acquired served me time and again. It's not bragging to call myself resilient, just like it's not bragging to tell people your personal best running times if you've worked for them. The knowledge that life puts many hills in front us is just as important as the awareness that I have what it takes to run up those hills. I've learned that, regardless of the outcome, I can run the marathon to the very last mile. There may be walk breaks along the way, or the path may change completely. Running, like infertility, builds you up, only to break you down.

17
NINE LIVES

Kat McNichol

"UM, SCOTT? I'M PREGNANT." I was hesitant, apologetic. I'd been trying to find a way to tell him all day.

"What? Shit! How did that happen?" My husband's reaction was what I had expected, but I was still disappointed.

"I'm not sure.... It sometimes happens with IUDs, I guess. It must, because I'm pregnant."

"I thought they were 99.9 percent effective."

"99.8 percent," I corrected. "Someone's gotta be in the 0.02 percent."

We stared at each other across the coffee table as I wrapped my hands protectively around my stomach.

"Aren't you even a little happy?" I asked. "You said you wanted a baby."

"Yes, but we're broke. We can't afford another kid."

"Scott, you always think we're broke. You're never going to say yes."

"It's not the right time, Kat."

"I'm not having an abortion."

"But, you said —"

"We were talking hypothetically. I really didn't think this would happen. I can't have another one."

I had my first abortion when I was 18 years old, just one week before I started university. A few months later, I had another. Then, in my early 20s, I had two daughters and learned what it really meant to love a child, so the thought of a third abortion — well, it was an impossible thought.

My face flushed hot as I held back my tears. I needed Scott to see my resolve. I could cry later. I spoke slowly and firmly. "I won't, Scott. No abortion. I'm sorry, but it is what it is. We're pregnant."

His body stilled and his back went rigid. Before I could say anything else, he stood up with a jerk and walked out, slamming the door hard behind him.

The next morning during my commute to work, I called my best friend.

"I'm pregnant," I said the second she answered.

"Kat? Did you say you're pregnant?"

"Yes, I'm pregnant." I felt tears looming again, and this time it was harder to hold them in.

Cassandra's voice softened. She's known me a long time and recognized the tremor in my words. "That's so great. I'm so happy for you. Are you excited?"

"Well, I was, but Scott's angry. He wants me to have an abortion, I think."

"What? Did he say that?"

"Not exactly. I cut him off before he could. He thinks we're broke."

I heard Cassandra snort. "He always thinks you're broke. You're not broke."

"I know."

"I think it'll be good for Scott. Break him out of his patterns a bit," she said.

"He'll be a good dad. He's already a good stepdad to my girls. He just —"

Cassandra interrupted. "He just can't handle change, that's all. He'll come around." Her voice was filled with conviction, and her certainty lessened my doubts.

"Kelly, Kat's pregnant," Cassandra yelled to her husband. I heard him mumble something in reply.

"What did he say?" I asked her.

"He says congratulations. Seriously, Kat, congrats. I know how much you've wanted another one."

"The doctor will see you now."

About time, I thought. I'd been sitting in the waiting room for nearly three hours.

In the examination room, the doctor, the same obstetrician I'd seen during my first pregnancy 10 years before, said, "So, you're pregnant."

He turned to the student intern he'd brought in with him. "She's got an IUD, but this still happens. I see this all the time."

Really? I thought. *You could have said that earlier.*

But the doctor seemed excited for me, and his excitement was infectious. By the time I left, I had a requisition for a blood test to confirm my pregnancy and a small plastic gift bag filled with coupons and pamphlets for new moms.

I'm pregnant. As I thought these words on the way back to my car, I realized that this was the first time I'd really felt their meaning. I clutched the little plastic gift bag in my hand and it swung rhythmically against my thigh: *I'm pregnant, I'm pregnant, I'm pregnant.*

Scott was waiting for me when I got home.

"How'd it go?" he asked in a quiet voice. I recognized the apologetic angle of his shoulders, his slight downward gaze.

"Fine," I said tersely, but I let my body take on a conciliatory posture.

"I'm sorry, Kat."

I nodded but stayed silent.

"I ... I'm just worried, you know, about money and work and my commute to Toronto and all the stress of that, and, I mean, can we afford for one of us to be home for a year?"

I shrugged, still standing at the door in my jacket, clutching my purse and little pregnancy bag.

"So ... we'll figure it out?" he asked.

I nodded again. "We always do," I replied.

"Okay. I'm sorry for how I reacted. I do really want to have a baby. "

"A girl, you said, right?" I asked, a smile tugging at the edge of my lips.

"Actually, I think a boy. There are too many girls already. I only have the fishes."

"The fish are probably girls, too." My giggle came out as a relieved sigh as a grin broke across my face.

Dropping my purse and jacket by the door, I flopped on the couch beside Scott. When he wrapped his arm around me, I snuggled into his side.

"I'm sorry, too," I said.

"For what? You didn't do anything."

"Oh, I'm just sorry in general, you know? I'm sorry life is so hard sometimes." After a pause, I asked in a tentative voice, "You want to see the pregnancy stuff the doctor gave me?"

"Sure."

"'Kay, give me a sec. I've had to pee the whole way home."

In the washroom, I saw tiny drops of blood on my underwear. *Sometimes that happens,* I reminded myself. *It's probably just implantation bleeding.*

Shaking away a slight sense of misgiving, I returned to the living room and spread the contents of the bag in front of Scott.

"Can I speak to Angela Kathleen McNichol, please?"

"Speaking," I replied.

"This is the OB nurse calling. We'd like to redo your pregnancy test. I have another requisition for you. Do you have a fax number?"

"Why, what's wrong?" I felt my heart speed up.

"The results of your first test show you're pregnant but the counts are low. How far along do you think you are?"

"Five weeks."

"Yeah, so the counts are low for five weeks. The doctor would like to retest."

"I've had some light bleeding the past couple days," I said with hesitation.

"Oh," she said sombrely. "Well."

That night, I started bleeding hard and the blood was filled with thick, heavy clots.

Sitting on the toilet watching the blood pour out, I cried all the tears I'd been holding back. The wretched sobbing that came out of me sounded like nothing I'd ever heard before.

"Kat, are you okay?" asked Scott through the bathroom door.

Through the mucus and tears that made it sound like I was drowning, I screamed, "No, I'm not okay, I'm not okay!"

"Let me in," yelled Scott, fear in his voice.

"No. Go away. I'm just … I'm not … I'm just not pregnant anymore!" Immediately, I felt the emptiness in those words, a deep pit in the base of my chest. Choking, I spit out, "Please, Scott, just leave me alone."

With Scott's support, I stopped using birth control, and six months later I was pregnant again. My family doctor ordered a blood test and an ultrasound. The blood test confirmed my pregnancy, and I went to the ultrasound eager to hear the baby's heartbeat.

"How far along are you?" asked the technician, wand in hand.

"About five weeks I think, but my periods haven't been consistent since my last pregnancy, so I don't know for sure."

"Well, I think you're not far enough along to see anything yet. Why did your doctor send you here so early?"

"Um, because of my previous difficulties, I guess?"

Nodding, she stared at the screen in front of her for a few more seconds before abruptly pulling the wand away.

"I'll schedule another appointment in two weeks and we'll try again."

It was a long two weeks.

When I returned, I had the same technician. I lay stiff with tension as she tried to find the baby in my belly. The room was quiet and her breathing sounded extra loud in the stillness, her exhalations timed with the panicky shriek in my head. I shut my eyes and took in deep gulps of air.

"You okay?" she asked with a glance in my direction.

"Yeah, yes, I'm fine, just nervous."

"Oh! Here's something. Finally."

But then she said nothing. The wand moved, she clicked her keyboard, but otherwise, silence. I waited, not breathing, but she just kept moving the wand and clicking.

"What?" I shouted, the word escaping before I could pull it back.

I felt her startled jump reverberate through my body. "I just see the yolk sac. It might be too early still to see anything more."

"No heartbeat?"

She shook her head. "Not yet."

"Do you feel pregnant?" my family doctor asked a week later as we reviewed my results.

I nodded quickly, yes.

"Okay. Well, we'll do another ultrasound and hope that this time there's a heartbeat. Hang in there."

But as I left, I thought about her question. *Do I feel pregnant? I feel like I want to feel pregnant, but that's not the same as feeling pregnant.*

This question weighed on me. It woke me at night from a deep sleep. *Do I feel pregnant?* The real answer was no. My breasts weren't sore, I wasn't nauseated, and I didn't have that sense of knowing that I'd had with my girls.

So I drove myself to the Fergus hospital. I couldn't face the crowded hospital in Guelph.

At triage, I said, "I'm pregnant, about eight weeks, but there hasn't been a heartbeat in any of the ultrasounds. I think I've miscarried." My voice was calm, formal.

Using a bedside ultrasound, the doctor confirmed what I already knew. "You've been holding on for a while now, eh?" he said.

I nodded.

"Well, we'll schedule a D&C and get this one out. You can try again." *Try again. Yes.*

Five months later, at a conference in San Diego, I realized my period was late. I found a drugstore, bought a pregnancy test, and in the hotel bathroom, watched while the positive pink line appeared. At the sight of that line, fear took root in my chest as I felt the months ahead stretch endlessly before me; time casts a long shadow when the timer keeps restarting.

I didn't call Scott that night. I'm not sure why. Maybe I was afraid to make it real. You can't lose something that isn't there.

The next day, I was leaving for a motorcycle trip in Baha, Mexico, with my CEO and one of my colleagues. While I waited in the hotel lobby for them to arrive, I finally called Scott.

"I'm pregnant."

"Oh, wow," he said. His voice was even, not excited, not upset. I held my breath and I think he held his. Then I heard him exhale.

"That's great, Kat." His voice cracked ever so slightly.

"Um, so, I've got to leave soon to go ride motorcycles in the mountains of Mexico," I said with a hint of drama. "Do you think it's okay if I go?"

"Yes, go. It can't hurt anything at this early stage, right?"

"No, probably not."

⌒⌒

"We train the military here," said our guide.

My colleague and CEO were impressed. I was terrified. I'm definitely not up to military fitness standards, and I doubt the soldiers are pregnant while they're training in the mountains.

We started off in a single-file convoy of two guides plus the three of us. I was second to last, with one of the guides riding behind me on a four-wheeler. I drove extra slow, and as we rode, I fell farther and farther behind the others. Every 20 minutes or so, they would stop so I could catch up. In my mirror, I saw the guide behind me impatiently swivelling from side to side. I felt bad for him — normally, I'd want to go faster, too, but not that day.

On the way down a steep slope the front wheel of my bike hit a rock at the wrong angle, and I suddenly found myself lying face down in the gravel, the wind knocked out of me. It was so quick; I was on the ground before I even realized I'd fallen.

The guide pulled up beside me, hopped off his bike and ran to my side.

"Shit, you okay?"

"I'm ... I can't do this," I groaned into the dirt.

"Do you want to ride my four-wheeler?" he asked.

"Maybe, yes, okay."

My CEO and colleague pulled up beside me as I brushed the dirt off my jacket and walked toward the four-wheeler.

"Hey, Kat, you're not giving up, are you?" yelled my colleague.

I stopped, looked over, and shook my head no. But I wanted to scream. I wanted to collapse in a ball at the side of the mountain path and just be still, to take in what I'd learned the night before.

I'm pregnant.

But instead, I resolved to get through the day, and then through the second day of this trip, with strength, because it wouldn't do to look weak in front of my CEO.

"Giving up?" I yelled as I ran to my fallen bike. "Hell no."

A couple weeks later, at seven weeks pregnant, I started spotting. An ultrasound showed there was an intact fetus but no heartbeat, and I was told again that bleeding at that stage was common and it might be too early to hear anything. I didn't believe them.

At my office a few days later, I suddenly started miscarrying with a vengeance.

I found myself back at the hospital, but this time they gave me morphine. By the time Scott arrived, I felt better.

A young doctor walked into my room and in a sober voice announced, "I've reviewed your ultrasound results, and I'm sorry, but this pregnancy is not viable."

Scott and I laughed.

Our laughter shocked the doctor, and in retrospect that makes sense, but we already knew we'd lost this pregnancy so his dramatic pronouncement struck us as funny.

Later that day, as I was rolled down the hall toward another D&C, my tears soaked the bed on either side of my head. The sensation was strange because other than these tears, I didn't feel like I was crying. The tears just came out on their own as if my body was crying without me.

⌘

Five months later, I was pregnant again.

When my obstetrician learned I'd lost my last two pregnancies without coming to see him, he got angry.

"Come to me," he nearly shouted before prescribing low-dose aspirin and progesterone pills to reduce the chances that I would miscarry again.

Right after filling my prescription for progesterone, Scott and I went to Tennessee. It was a business trip for him, but we combined it with a few days of vacation. While he was at his first day of business meetings, I took my first progesterone pill and within hours I was vomiting.

From the floor of the hotel bathroom, I called my obstetrician and learned that sometimes women react badly to progesterone when it's taken orally. He suggested I insert the pills vaginally instead.

We visited Ruby Falls in Chattanooga on that trip. It was the last day of our vacation and I was feeling better. The falls were magnificent. After a long walk through a tight stalactite-filled pathway through interconnected caves, we arrived in a massive cavern created by a breathtaking underground waterfall. Trying to capture some of the magic in that cavern, I made a wish for my baby.

⌘

At seven weeks along, I went for an ultrasound, and it was the kind of ultrasound I remembered having when I was pregnant with my daughters. The ultrasound technician chatted while she scanned my stomach and then turned the screen to show me the bloodlines flashing. She turned a dial and the sound of galloping filled the room.

"It's wonderful, that sound, isn't it?" she asked and I nodded, speechless.

"All the stages are so fun to see. I especially like ten weeks when the baby looks like a little gingerbread man." She giggled thinking about it.

"I'm looking forward to that stage," I whispered, still staring at the pulsing colours on the screen.

I left with an ultrasound photo, with the word *baby* printed on the front.

"I can see it in your hips already," said Scott. His eyes seemed to glow as he looked at me.

At 10 weeks pregnant, I walked to the park with my mom. It was cold and I was wearing a rainbow-coloured knit hat with a big pompom on top and flaps that hung past my ears on either side.

"You look cute in that hat," said Mom with a smile.

I nodded, but tucked my arms around me with a shrug.

"Are you okay?" she asked.

"Something's wrong, Mom. I can feel it."

"With the baby?" Her voice was sharp.

"I think so. I don't feel pregnant. I did before, but I don't anymore." I thought about what it meant the last time I didn't feel pregnant.

"Honey, you're just anxious because of the others. Your ultrasound was fine this time. You're fine, the baby's fine, okay?"

I nodded. My mom's reassurance made me feel better. I resolved not to worry.

My 12-week ultrasound appointment took forever to arrive. Waiting was painful. The appointment was scheduled for the same day I was to leave for a conference in Indianapolis. My plan was to get the ultrasound, go to my follow-up appointment with my obstetrician, then drive to Detroit, where I'd spend the night, finishing the drive the next morning. I packed a suitcase for my trip.

I felt good that day, confident. I wore a loose hot-pink blouse and a pair of stylish maternity jeans.

The technician at this ultrasound was a young man. I'd never had a male ultrasound technician before.

"Do I need to put on a gown?" I asked him.

"No, that's okay, just hop up here, lift your shirt, and slide your pants down to your hips."

He tucked white paper into the top of my pants to keep them clean from the gel. "Hopefully this baby isn't too active. We've got a lot of pictures to take today," he said as he adjusted the paper around me.

But as soon as he put the wand on my stomach, he went silent. His breathing was loud, like the previous technician's. The clicking was loud and the wand dug into my stomach.

After a few minutes, he wiped me clean.

"Okay, all done. The doctor will give you your results."

"But what are they?"

"I'm sorry, I can't give you results. I'm not allowed to."

"Okay, but usually you guys show me the heartbeat, give me an ultrasound photo. You can't do that?"

"No," he whispered, and I felt the blood drain from my face.

"You have to tell me," I said, the sound of a sob in the back of my throat. "I already know but please, please just say it."

"Promise you won't tell anyone I told you?" he asked in a stage whisper.

"Yes, I promise."

"I'm sorry, there's no heartbeat."

I nodded then quickly pulled my maternity pants up over my belly, jumped off the bed, and fled.

The ultrasound office was in a mall in downtown Guelph. I called Scott from the first bench I saw. The phone rang in my ear as people streamed around me, but I felt so alone, I might as well have been on a desert island.

"Hello?"

"Scott. Scott."

"Kat?"

"There's no heartbeat."

"What? Oh no, Kat, why?"

"I don't know," I shouted, then catching myself, I said in a quiet rush, "I have my follow-up appointment with the obstetrician now. I'll go to that. Maybe he can tell me. The technician wouldn't tell me anything else. I made him tell me about the heartbeat. I've probably ruined his day."

"Who cares about his day, Kat. Take care of *yourself*, okay? Do you want me to come?"

"Not yet. Let me go to the doctor, then I'll call you. I'm not going to the conference though."

"Obviously."

"I need to email work and tell them."

"Work can wait. They think you're driving anyway. Tell them tomorrow."

"Okay, okay. I gotta go. My appointment … "

"Okay, bye."

"Love you."

"Love you, too."

From the parking lot of my obstetrician's office, I called the nurse.

"I'm outside. I just came from my ultrasound appointment and there's no heartbeat." I felt my voice shake on the words. "I don't want to sit in the waiting room, so when it's my turn, can you just call and I'll come up?"

"Oh, I'm sorry, the doctor's not here today."

"But I had an appointment."

"I rescheduled all his appointments for today."

"You didn't reschedule mine."

"I must have missed you. Sorry about that. I can reschedule your appointment to early next week. Does that work for you?"

"Um, no, that doesn't work for me. Did you hear me? There's no heartbeat."

She was silent for a minute, and then said, "I'm sorry. There's nothing I can do for you now."

"Okay, ah, thank you. Never mind then." And I hung up.

Sitting in my car, I stared at the phone in my hand, wondering what I should do. The one thing I knew for sure was that I didn't want to hold this dead baby inside me anymore. I wanted it out.

Pulling myself together, I went to the Guelph hospital.

In triage, the nurse put her hand on mine as I sobbed. "Please get it out. Please, please get it out."

"I'm taking you straight back. We're full but there's an inner waiting room. Are you in pain?"

"No, I feel nothing. Just … nothing."

"Okay, wait here. We'll get you into a room as soon as we can. It won't be long."

In the inner waiting room, I looked around me at the other people waiting. Most looked sick but some stared at me with interest.

To get away from their eyes, I went to the washroom and there I found blood in my underwear. I called Scott. "Why am I bleeding now? I haven't bled at all in twelve weeks."

"You're really stressed right now, Kat. Stress is powerful. It's probably kick-started things."

"Yeah, yes, that makes sense. Come now, okay, Scott? I can't be alone."

"We've had your results sent over from the ultrasound clinic. The fetus is no longer viable. We're scheduling you for a D&C."

"But how long ago did it die?"

"You want to know that? Okay, it's measuring eight weeks and one day. It probably passed at nine or ten weeks. It gets smaller over time after passing."

Oh, God. It's disintegrating.

"Okay," I whispered. "Thank you."

At home, as I unpacked maternity clothes from my suitcase for the trip I never took, I asked Scott to tell his family what had been happening.

"Can you just email them and let them know? Otherwise, they'll ask us about babies again."

That October, a few weeks after my fourth miscarriage, Scott's mom came from Vancouver for Thanksgiving and for Scott's birthday. During the visit, I was sitting alone on the couch in our living room when Scott's sister sat beside me and handed me her phone.

"Look at this new app I just got."

On her phone was a pink calendar app.

"I don't understand." I said, smiling.

"It's a pregnancy calendar."

"Oh." I paused. "You're pregnant? Well, that's ... I mean ... congratulations. I'm so happy for you."

She nodded. Looking down, I registered the slight swell of her stomach for the first time.

We sat awkwardly together for a few more minutes as I tried to act happy, but sadness swelled and swelled until I felt like I would choke. I carried that choking feeling all day. It was Scott's birthday.

As we waited for a table at Turtle Jack's, Scott's sister told my daughters that she was pregnant.

"Oh, wow, you're pregnant?" said 11-year-old Asia.

"That's so cool," said 10-year-old Allie. "We get a new cousin."

I listened silently, trying not to look too upset.

"Mommy?" said Allie, turning to me. "When are you going to have another baby?"

"Yeah!" said Asia, "I want a baby sister. You said you wanted another baby someday. What's taking so long?"

It felt like I'd been punched. "Girls, I'm just, I guess I'm not ready yet. Can we talk about this later? Now's not the best time, okay?"

But before I'd even finished my sentence, they were gone, bouncing off to the next conversation. I was left standing with Scott's mom and sister, their eyes filled with sympathy.

"It's okay," I said. "I'm fine, no worries. I think our table's ready."

But the next day, I couldn't get out of bed even though Scott's mom was waiting to spend the day with us.

"Scott, I can't, I just can't," I sobbed from under the blanket.

I felt like I was smothered in sadness. Even the blanket felt heavy, and the thought of the day ahead, of being friendly and acting like I was happy — it was all too much.

"Kat, it's okay. I'll take my mom and the girls to the mall. Okay? Does that work?"

"Yes, yes, okay, yes."

I cuddled deep into my blanket and let myself fall into a heavy sleep.

Four months later, a few days before leaving for a conference in Baltimore, I learned I was pregnant again.

Before I left, the obstetrician had blood drawn to confirm my pregnancy.

"Are you certain about your dates?" the OB nurse asked when she called with my results.

"Yes, absolutely positive. Scott and I only had sex once this whole month. We're a little shell-shocked from all the miscarriages."

"I understand. The levels are low, though, for four weeks."

"Oh, so it's happening again, then."

"No, not necessarily. It's really early still. Have faith."

"Sure, okay."

The next morning I woke up feeling slightly nauseated, something I hadn't felt since I was pregnant with my younger daughter. I allowed myself to feel a tiny glimmer of hope.

That evening, my colleagues and I went to a restaurant on the wharf in Baltimore. All evening, I poured my drinks into the toilet as I watched the rest of my colleagues get drunk.

I'm pregnant, I'm pregnant, I'm pregnant ran like a mantra in my head.

I herded the group of them along the wharf after dinner, until we came to what looked like a clown car painted like a police car.

"Is it actually a police car?" one of them asked.

"Yeah, that's what they use to patrol the wharf," replied another.

"Let's get in it."

"Guys, that's not a good idea," I said, but three of them were already climbing into the car.

"Hey, seriously, not a good plan," I shouted, just as a police officer walked around the edge of the building.

The group in the car saw him and froze. He pointed to a camera above the police car as the three clambered out. "Sorry, sorry, sorry, sorry."

"Let's go, now," I told them, and I led the group back toward the restaurant we'd just come from to flag down a cab.

"Wow, Kat," one of them slurred. "You can really hold your alcohol."

Back in Canada, I took another blood test and this time my hormone levels were high.

"So far, so good," the OB nurse told me.

At seven weeks, the ultrasound technician found a heartbeat, but although I was relieved, I chose not to take an ultrasound photo home with me.

My goal was to be as calm as possible, to keep my stress levels low so my body would stay healthy, but at eight weeks and one day, I saw blood in my underwear.

I called Scott on my way to the hospital.

"I'm bleeding," I told him quietly.

"Oh. Do you want me to come?" he asked.

"No, it's okay; we both know how this goes. Just get me when it's over."

In the hospital's ultrasound room, I lay with my face turned away from the screen.

"Which number of pregnancies is this?" asked the technician.

"My ninth," I replied in a voice that sounded like it belonged to someone else. I could tell she was shocked.

"How many living?" she asked.

"Two."

I didn't tell her about my abortions.

After a long pause, she said, "Well, you're persistent."

I nodded, still staring at the wall.

I felt nothing as I lay there waiting for her to finish. I expected to go back to the emergency ward where the doctor would tell me he was scheduling a D&C, but that's not what happened.

"There's a heartbeat," the technician announced as she turned the screen toward me.

"What?"

"There's a heartbeat," she repeated.

Stunned, tears welled in my eyes. "I don't know what to do with that," I said, and even to myself I sounded broken.

She very gently wiped my stomach clean.

"But why am I bleeding?" I choked out.

"The doctor will tell you that part, but don't worry, it's not a big deal." It turned out to be a small uterine hemorrhage of little significance.

A few days later, at nine weeks pregnant, I left for a business trip to Japan. In the upside-down time zone on the other side of the globe, I was nauseated the whole time. It felt wonderful to be nauseated like that. Nausea was good. Nausea meant this pregnancy was surviving.

Scott came with me to my 12-week ultrasound. I'd always done ultrasounds on my own, but this time I was afraid to be alone in case the news was bad again. In the waiting room before my appointment, I sat at the edge of my seat and every muscle in my body jittered.

"Kat, calm down."

"I'll calm down when it's over, Scott."

But when the technician came to get me, she said, "He can come in at the end." So Scott waited outside while I went in alone.

After a lot of clicking, she smiled and said, "Okay, I'll go get your husband now," and I released the breath I'd been holding.

Scott's eyes lit up at the sight of the person-shaped image on the screen.

"You got yourself a little Olympian in there," said the technician.

Afterward, Scott told me, "I was scared waiting alone. The way you were so nervous before you went in, and then it took so long for her to come get me."

I nodded. I knew the feeling.

"But as soon as I saw the baby swimming around like that... Everything's going to be okay this time."

"Don't, Scott. Don't get so excited yet, okay?"

Every morning, I'd leave for work, buy coffee at Planet Bean, vomit into my empty coffee cup from the day before, and then drink the new coffee I'd just bought. I became adept at driving and vomiting at the same time, but each time it happened, I welcomed it. It was a daily reminder that this pregnancy was going well.

I vomited every morning until I was 17 weeks pregnant and only stopped vomiting after I stopped the progesterone pills, but by then I could feel the baby moving inside me.

At my 20-week ultrasound, we brought my daughters along with us and hoped we weren't tempting fate with their optimism.

"What do you think it's going to be, Scott?" asked Asia.

"A girl," said Scott. "It would be nice if it was a boy, though."

"No way," Allie shouted. "Yuck. It has to be a girl. What do boys even wear?"

"Boy clothes, silly," snorted Asia. "Mommy, what do you think?"

"I think a girl. We always have girls in our family."

"Yeah, I think a girl, too," said Asia.

"It's a boy," said the technician.

We stared at the screen in shocked silence.

"Is that okay?" the technician asked.

"Yes, of course it's okay," I said. "I just didn't know I could make boys."

"How do you know it's a boy?" asked Allie.

"See this?" she pointed. "That's his penis."

"Oh my gosh, it's bigger than his head," said Asia, her words reverberating against the walls of the little room.

The technician exploded with laughter and then so did the rest of us, and as we all laughed, for the first time I thought, *It's going to be okay.*

And it was. Our son, Jake, was born 18 long weeks later, on September 10, 2014.

Even as all this was happening, life went on, though at times it felt like nothing would be normal again. There's a line by T.S. Eliot that I think puts it best: "At the still point of the turning world. Neither flesh nor fleshless / Neither from nor toward; at the still point, there the dance is."

18
SIDELINE GRIEF

Kyle Miller

SINCE I CAN REMEMBER, I have wanted to have a family of my own: a wife and a few kids. I'm an optimist at heart, but for some reason, when it came to kids and pregnancies, I always had doubts. My mother was open about the struggles she went through when she was trying to create a family. She had two miscarriages before she had my brother and me. I used to say to her that I was glad it had happened, because I wouldn't have been born otherwise. Looking back, I was clearly young and didn't understand the gravity of the experience my mother and father had gone through.

Fast-forward a few decades. I'm living with a beautiful dog and I meet the woman of my dreams, Erica. We renovate her grandfather's house and move in, get married, and get pregnant, all within two years. I absolutely can't wait to be a daddy. We find out about the pregnancy on our way to my friend's wedding, and by the end of the night, everyone knows Erica's expecting. I know everyone says you should wait until after 12 weeks for the announcement, but I'm so excited and I can't keep secrets.

Erica's pregnancy proceeds as expected: cravings, some nausea, and, of course, moodiness we blamed on the hormones. It isn't until she is 12 weeks pregnant that I start to get nervous, and my mother's experiences with her pregnancies begin to replay in my mind. Although I always thought I would be prepared for a miscarriage while making my own family, the truth is that I'm not. I want this baby more than anything, and I already have so much love devoted to him. I hold my breath until we are given the all-clear that everything is happening as it should be.

I'm not sure how interested most men are in their partner's pregnancy, but for me it was never a question that I would be involved as much as possible. The second I see the word *pregnant* on the overpriced pregnancy test, in my mind I'm already a daddy. I download a pregnancy app on my smartphone so that I can follow along closely as the weeks fly by. My baby boy is the size of a lima bean, an apple, then an eggplant. It's just so exciting. I paint the nursery and assemble new furniture. We have a gender-reveal party and a baby shower for friends and family. The due date for our boy, my birthday, comes and goes, and two days later Erica wakes me up to tell me she is bleeding. I immediately go into internal panic mode where all I can think of is the worst outcome possible.

Externally, I am calm and collected. I take Erica to the hospital to make sure things are okay. She gets admitted right away. After a quick exam, the doctor tells us that Erica is three centimetres dilated and she will be staying at the hospital to deliver the baby.

On June 5, 2013, it takes 17 intense hours for my handsome little man, Hudson Miller, to join us. I am finally a dad. Nothing in my life has prepared me for what's just happened. I have never held a baby before in my life, but when the nurse hands my new son to me, it feels so natural. His smell, his warmth, and the little noises he makes give me peace and fill my heart with so much love.

Our little man is just over a year old when Erica and I decide to start trying to have another baby. Both of us come from families with two children, and we have always planned on the same family dynamic. After trying for a few months, Erica becomes pregnant once again in the summer of 2014. Because Erica's pregnancy with Hudson was so smooth, I assume this one will be the same.

At the end of the summer, we decide to go for a little getaway and we rent a cottage for a week up north. Erica is about nine weeks pregnant. We relish this chance to spend time with our little family of three before growing into a family of four. And then the world stops.

The day before we are supposed to go home, Erica begins to spot. When she tells me, my heart sinks. This is it. What I had always thought would happen is happening. I do everything I can to reassure Erica that it will be okay. Google tells us that this can sometimes happen and it might be normal. Google also presents some horrifying facts I decide to withhold from Erica since I don't want to upset her further. In my heart I know what's happening, but I have to be strong for her. I have to be positive. I know she's already freaking out and thinking the worst. All I want to do is comfort her and take the pain away, but I can't. And it's killing me.

We go to the emergency room the day we get back home. A doctor, lacking any training in human interaction, comes into the room, and with no emotion tells us there is no heartbeat. The baby stopped growing weeks earlier. I don't remember his words exactly, but they are heartless, and I want to punch him in the face for how he carelessly tells us our baby is dead. Erica understandably breaks down crying, and the doctor seems confused as to why she is so upset. Somehow I manage to ignore him and maintain my composure so that I can be strong for my wife. But inside, knowing our baby is gone, I am crushed.

The next few days and weeks, we function on autopilot. Erica and I try to avoid talking about the miscarriage by keeping busy with Hudson and giving him our full attention. It isn't until I have time alone that I reflect on what happened and allow myself to break down. I've just lost a child. I'll never get to hold my baby in my arms and sing them a lullaby. The pregnancy app tells us that our baby was the size of a raspberry when we lost them, so that's what we decide to call the baby.

My mom told me how my dad never got over their miscarriages. He used to look at his thumb while he drove and he would cry because that was the size of one of their children when they lost them. I find myself doing the same thing. On longer drives I get a glimpse of my hand on the steering wheel and the image of my child I never got to meet floods my thoughts, and I can't get it out of my head. Sometimes I ugly cry.

I'm lucky that I come from a family that is open and honest. We aren't the Brady Bunch by any stretch, but we were taught to embrace our emotions, including having a good cry if need be (though my crying was more often than not caused by my getting in trouble and being sent to my room). I was never taught to feel shame about crying in the way that so many boys are told that crying is for babies and girls. Allowing myself to cry when we lost the baby was cathartic and helped me to release the grief I was feeling, a little bit each time. I cried with Erica when we found out, I cried with my mother when I told her, and I still cry now and then when I'm in deep thought and think about our loss.

Despite the fact that we are still living with the devastation of losing Raspberry, we want so badly to give Hudson a sibling. A couple more months of trying to conceive and we are pregnant with what I learn people call a rainbow baby — a pregnancy after the loss of a baby. This time I'm not nearly as confident. I am terrified and I know Erica is, too.

I'm not the eager dad I was with the other pregnancies, and I don't tell anyone about it except for some of my co-workers I'm close with. But things seem to be going well as we approach the 12-week ultrasound. We breathe a little sigh of relief that we've made it this far.

Our ultrasound is scheduled for the Friday before Family Day weekend. We plan to announce the great news to our families at dinner.

We arrive at the clinic, a different one than from our previous ultrasounds. Erica goes into the room to have the ultrasound while I sit patiently in the waiting room. I'm a little nervous, but I figure that's just part of the excitement and it will settle once I get to go in and see for myself that everything is okay.

But I don't get to go in and see the ultrasound this time. No nurse comes out to get me like they did before, and that's when I know something is wrong. When Erica walks out of the exam room, the look on her face makes me more nervous. She hands me the picture and says she thinks something is off. She explains that the nurse's reactions and facial expressions were concerning. I try to assure her that it's all in her head and that the nurse is probably just one who does her job and doesn't really like to interact with patients all that much. I love my wife, but she is one of those people who look for risks or cons in any situation, so my response to her reactions always tends to be optimistic.

I still have hope, and I figure it can't hurt for Erica to have some as well.

Even when we come home and put the picture of our new baby on the fridge, Erica can't help but compare the ultrasound picture of Hudson to this baby's and point out differences she sees, like a shortened neck and different legs. I don't really notice a huge difference and chalk it up to the photo being at a different angle.

That night we receive a phone call from our family doctor's office. They want us to come in the next day. They don't say why, but Erica immediately thinks the worst. "They never call at night for good news," she says.

As much as I know she's right, I want to hold on to hope. I think of all the possible reasons why they could be calling and reassure Erica it will be okay. I don't know what else to do.

The rest of the night is pretty solemn. We don't speak much. We watch TV, but there is so much tension and emotion in the room, it's almost unbearable. We are both in our own worlds, going over every possibility in our heads of what could be wrong with the baby.

I try to hold on to what few facts I have: We heard a heartbeat. We have a picture of our baby. *We're going to be fine.*

The next day, my mother comes over to babysit Hudson while we go to the doctor. We tell her that we have a financial meeting, because we still haven't told our families we're pregnant. I'm in the exam room with Erica when the doctor comes in. I'll never forget the look on her face as she shut the door behind her. Right away, she says that she's sorry for what we are about to go through.

She tells us our baby has some abnormalities: stunted growth and thickness in the neck. We are devastated. I assume what I think is my role, to listen to the doctor and write down all of the follow-up information, while also trying to console my wife, who is beside herself after the first few words come out of the doctor's mouth. It feels like the first time, when we lost Raspberry, only worse. I'm outwardly calm and somehow hold in the absolute devastation of what is happening inside of me.

Although I know I can express myself if I want to, if I need to, I want to be strong for my wife. I want her not to have to worry about me, because I know that while this is devastating for me, it's going to be worse for her.

We need to have a more detailed ultrasound, as well as other tests, to understand what is going on.

After we get home, I walk over to my mom, give her a hug, and let myself cry, not letting go. She asks over and over what's wrong, but I can't speak. After staying like that for a long time, I finally get the words out: "Erica's pregnant, but something's wrong with our baby."

Over the next few days, Erica and I go over every possibility of what could be wrong with our baby. We talk about raising a child with an exceptionality and loving them regardless. The hardest part of these days is knowing our baby is not okay, but not knowing why.

Finally the day comes for us to go to the hospital and have the ultrasound, blood work, and whatever other barrage of tests done. Afterward, we meet with a specialized genetics counsellor who breaks the news to us. Our baby has osteogenesis imperfecta type III. This is not a viable pregnancy. She has broken ribs and a broken femur, and her skull is not formed. In that moment we are dealt two blows in one. That we are having a baby girl. And that we won't be able to have her on this earth.

At this, I have no words of hope or optimism left. I have no words of encouragement for Erica. I have no words of encouragement for myself. I am just devastated. And I give in to it.

A week or so later, Erica and I are back in the hospital to be induced. Erica doesn't want to be bothered during the procedure, so I wait on the sidelines, again not knowing what to say or do. I just sit there. I participate in my own way, by praying to God to comfort Erica and to take care of my baby girl.

Erica gives birth to our daughter a few hours after being induced. The nurses wrap the baby up in a cute little dress, and I hold her and cry. She is so small, fitting neatly into the palm of my hand. We ask to have the chaplain at the hospital say a blessing for her, which helps ease some of the pain. We name her Reese.

After some genetic testing is done on Reese's remains to see if it is likely to happen in a subsequent pregnancy, we have her cremated. I have a necklace made with her name on it that holds some of her ashes so that she will always be with me. I have a bracelet made for Erica as well. The nurses at the hospital gave us a card with Reese's two little footprints on it.

We receive inconclusive evidence from Reese's genetic testing. But we decide to start trying for another baby. As much as I want another child, this time around I don't have the same emotional connection as before. Erica uses ovulation sticks to get the timing right, and I'm used for what I bring to the table. When we have sex, it isn't as natural as it was prior to our losses. The added pressure of wanting to conceive mixed with the fear of becoming pregnant again and the possibility of loss make it all feel like a job that needs doing.

It takes longer for us to get pregnant this time, but in the summer of 2015, we find out we are expecting again. I express my excitement but distance myself from feeling connected to the life that is happening inside Erica. I'm so broken from the last two pregnancies that I can't invest my heart into this one, not yet.

Erica is doing an amazing job with this pregnancy, just like with all the others, but I can tell she is being extra careful. It's like she feels that if anything happens to this baby, it's not going to be because of anything she did. She tries to get me interested in feeling the baby kick or asks me if I see the baby move, but my responses are less than enthusiastic. I touch her abdomen and reply with a sullen, "Oh yeah, cool," or I glance over a second too late and say, "No, I missed it," pretending to be disappointed but actually feeling relieved.

When she asks me about my lack of interest in the pregnancy, I lie and say it's just because I'm too preoccupied with Hudson to think about all the baby stuff like I did before. But since I'm usually the happy and optimistic one, my disinterest does not sit well with Erica, no matter the reason. Eventually we have a conversation about why I'm acting withdrawn from the baby, and even though she understands and respects my perspective, I can tell she is annoyed by it. I get why. If I feel like this — scared of heartbreak, of getting too attached — imagine how she feels. And she's right. It's selfish, and I'm lucky that I have the prerogative to stay detached, since I'm not the one with the baby inside of me. But it's a mechanism that kicks in automatically, almost without my will, to protect me. Because I can't go through the heartbreak again.

The time comes. We are in hospital, 18 hours into labour, and the heart-rate monitor drops. I hear someone say, "The baby is in distress. We're going to have to take drastic measures."

I can barely stand from the fear that overwhelms me. *Not again. We're so close.*

I pray repeatedly for God not to let anything happen to the baby or Erica. I hold my breath, my chest pounding, and wait. Finally, I hear the most beautiful sound of a baby cry and let myself exhale. My baby girl

is finally here, and she is healthy and crying. All the love I've been holding back comes pouring out of me. In an instant, I fall so in love with
my daughter. And more than that, I fall in love with my wife. I am so
proud of her for shouldering the lion's share of our burden, for putting
her body through what it needed to go through for our family to now,
finally, be complete.

We name her Leighton.

I always thought the open conversations my parents had with me about
miscarriage and infant loss would prepare me if my family were ever to go
through it. I thought it was just something that happens to people and, because of that, there was a good chance it would happen to my family as well.
But to this day, I haven't been more wrong or naive about anything in my life.

As a man, a husband, and a father, I didn't expect that I would feel the
intensity of grief for my babies that I did. I didn't expect to feel as if my heart
had been ripped out of my chest. Because of what I've been through, I honestly and truly feel for the women who experience child loss in any form. Even
after witnessing it, I can't imagine what they have to go through physically
and emotionally when they lose a baby. They get to experience a physical
bond with their baby only to have that taken away in an instant. As a man,
I didn't get that physical connection with my babies, but to the best of my
ability, I know that the grief I felt was right up there with my wife's. These
experiences of loss were the most challenging of my life.

Other than the obvious part of losing our babies, having to take on the
role of counsellor, when that's what I needed, too, was probably the hardest
part. Right or wrong, I felt my grief needed to be put on the sideline so I could
focus on what was most important to me, which was the well-being of my
wife. As a man, I felt that it would have been selfish to ask my wife to console
me when we were going through the same thing but she was the one carrying
the baby. In hindsight, I could have and should have opened up more about
how I was feeling. It might have helped both of us in our journey and grieving.

I feel that men, unfortunately, aren't encouraged to seek counsel from
others when it comes to a partner's miscarriage. Everyone always seems to

care about the mental health of the woman, leaving the man with a compulsory "How you doing?" as comfort, and little else.

I'm lucky I was able to connect with and confide in some co-workers who helped me through my loss, but I never really got a chance to connect with another dad who shared the same perspective as me, which I think could have made all the difference. I'm sharing my story in the hope that it might help even one man to know he is not alone in his grief, that it is real, and that it's okay to talk about it.

We finally have the family we always dreamed of and life is beautifully crazy. We still count our blessings every day. We have two healthy, happy, and wild kids at home who we will love with every breath we take for the rest of our lives. I can't begin to explain how proud I am of my wife for how she handled two difficult losses and still managed to produce an angel of a baby afterward. Being on the sidelines and watching her during these four pregnancies has changed my perspective. She is the strongest person I know, and I've gained a whole new appreciation and love for her that I didn't have before we had kids.

Although we are moving forward as a family at a crazy pace, I never want to forget about the past or about our babies we never got to raise. I don't want to be ashamed about talking about our losses. I decided to get tattoos of both Leighton and Hudson, and within their names are Reese's footprints that the nurse gave to us on the card. Our babies will always be a part of us, and I'll never forget the feelings of joy they gave me.

With time, healing has come, but there will always be a part of me that will miss the babies I never got to take home. I will always wonder what they would have been like. I know they are watching down on us, and in some ways I look forward to the day our family of four on earth can be reunited as a family of six on the other side.

19

IN THE SPACE BETWEEN

Charlotte Dobo

I ALWAYS THOUGHT IT WOULD BE bigger when it happened, you know? I thought maybe it would be accompanied by a cacophonous roar that signals the end times.

I imagined that most horrifying of horrifying things happening to me, even in an abstract way; it was ominous. I thought it would feel like buildings burning to the ground in impossible-to-fight fires and people screaming, wild-eyed in the streets, holding their heads in their hands and desperately searching the faces of strangers for solace. I thought I'd be helpless against all of it when it did happen, whenever that was.

I thought, if it ever happened — and it could — because we all know a person who knows a person who *it* did happen to — it would ruin me. I thought that the conflicted feelings I was sure to feel would intertwine in the air like vapours and that they would seep into the walls and the cloth of the sofa and the sheets of my bed and that I would never, ever, feel the same again. That is, of course, if *it* ever happened.

I'm a worrier — I have been since as far back as I can remember. But pregnancy brought with it this whole new world of worries, ones I had never had to carry before.

Naturally, during my first of two healthy, very uneventful pregnancies (which yielded big, bouncing baby boys), I worried about every single thing: strange twinges of pain, shallow breathing, miscarriage. I worried about dying during labour. I worried about an emergency Caesarean section. I worried about blood transfusions. I read all the books ever published and the entirety of the internet and they fed my fears. During the first and second trimesters, I silently counted down, week by week, based on a chart I found somewhere, its accuracy never clear, ticking each passing week off like some kind of *fait accompli* — because each week would bear a reduced risk of miscarriage, and then of stillbirth. I would tally each passing week, taking a deep breath as I inched closer to the third trimester, the time when even if you go into premature labour, the odds of your baby surviving are in your favour.

Once I was into weeks 30 and higher, when my anxiety should have eased, I catastrophized. I worried about a loss so tremendous that it would stop all the clocks, throw the solar system out of orbit. As I imagined it, the loss would come out of nowhere and smash into my life like a wayward transport truck slipping on the most treacherous of ice. So when I lost her, when I lost Florence — that was her name — I was surprised. Shocked, even, at the way I lost her. She left me like a slow-burning candle that had burned down to the last of the wick and lingered, even then, for too long. Burning impossibly but still burning, somehow. After that, the loneliness that set in was crushing. I was surrounded by things, my sons, my pets, my co-workers, my friends, but nothing could fill the deep emptiness that came when she left.

After my separation from my sons' father, I had jumped, head first and flat on my face, into a bad relationship that should never have been. I was lonely, and someone wanted me, and that felt like enough. But he treated me like garbage — I mean, in ways I would never dream of treating another living being. He saw my role of mother as some kind of black mark against me, not as something that effectively made me the person I am, the person he claimed to love. There was abuse and violence of all sorts, and in many ways I'm still very far away from a place where it feels safe to talk about any of it.

A friend of mine put it best. When I explained that he had treated me like shit the entire time we were together, she said, "But sometimes that's really attractive, for whatever reason, when you're in a bad place."

I had never thought of it like that, but she was so right that it hurt. I felt shame for ever having put myself in that position. I know well enough that abuse and violence are cyclical and that the very best, smartest, most aware of us get caught up in it unwittingly. I felt sadness for all the misplaced efforts I had made. For opening my heart at all to something so vile.

My reaction to the pregnancy, which was very unexpected, was one of dismay and anger. I was so upset because I knew, without a doubt, that there was only one outcome: I would eventually work up the courage to tell him, and he would tell me to "get rid of it." News of the pregnancy, which I admittedly waited too long to share with him, was poorly received. It was my fault. I had done it on purpose. I was the type of woman who got pregnant to collect child support. Everything he could think to say in his strategy of emotional attrition was said. He threw down each accusation, each biting judgment, like a bloody hammer on my life. He told me to do whatever I wanted, but never to expect anything from him.

We didn't talk after that. And even though his brand of love was like a poison, in the days after that I had no one. No one to talk to, no one I felt I could tell.

My other reaction to the impending arrival of a third baby, as a single parent, was to set aside my grief and terror at the multitude of what-ifs, as if I were putting them all on a shelf to deal with one day, and to instead do the most practical thing I could think of: scour the internet for baby things. All the things I'd since sold or given to my little sister, who was expecting a baby just a few months before this one was due. I quickly assembled what I could and stuffed it all into a closet in my tiny house. As I thumbed through bags of impossibly small second-hand shirts and sleepers and mismatched socks, I thought, *This isn't what you planned, it's true, but you're going to be okay.*

The short, blurry ensuing weeks revealed that this unexpected baby was also unexpectedly unwell. They used phrases like *genetic abnormality* and *deficiencies not compatible with life* to try to explain it to me. Too many words to ascribe to the most impossible of impossible situations. Too many words to say, "It's over."

All of the routine, administrative things that took place after this revelation are a blur of waivers and blood tests, ultrasounds, genetic counsellors, and psychologists. Life swirled around me, and I was at the mercy of everyone's schedule. I recall walking my son to preschool and, without fail each morning, a neighbour, a woman whose name I didn't know but who I recognized, would stop me to tell me I looked "so sad." It was written on my face by then: this woman has a dying baby in her body. Be patient. Be kind.

I was 21.5 weeks along when it happened. In the few weeks during which I lived thinking a healthy baby was en route and that she would blow a hole through my life, I had come to terms with the idea of her. Conceptually, we would be okay. I was 34 and thought maybe it was my body's way of offering me one last kick at the can. I had always said I wanted three kids, before I had any. Except now I had two boys at home, and we were on our own, and this was never how I had mapped my life out by any stretch of the imagination.

I arrived at the hospital a bit late for my induction appointment. There had been so much traffic on the way to the hospital; I thought, *Of course there is.* I remember how it felt to cross the threshold from sidewalk to hospital and that I had done the very same thing with my other two kids, not so long ago that I had forgotten. Except when you're coming to deliver a baby who will never make it, you go to a different floor. You won't make friends with the other lady trying to keep her shit together in a gown, clutching those railings in the maternity ward. You'll be on your own. Where you've already felt like you've been for so long.

After 48 hours, six rounds of induction medication, 12 hours of labouring, and an hour of pushing, she was gone. Never a breath of air outside. Never a moment to look into her eyes and honour the 21.5 weeks we had spent together.

I spent hours after that crying, in a pit of loneliness that stung. How would I ever feel the same after this? How could I?

Like the births of my two boys, her birth came with all the things: it was rigorous and exhausting and emotional and defeating and so, so painful. In her case, after waiting six hours for the placenta to deliver unsuccessfully, I underwent a dilation and curettage (D&C) as well. I was so emotionally exhausted after hours of induction meds, progress checks, and pushing. Of thinking the doctors and nurses weaving in and out of the room saying "Progress check" were misinformed; nothing here was progressing to any good place, to any sort of completion.

I pleaded with them not to put me to sleep for the D&C. I panicked that after all that had happened, I would die on the table and never see my boys again. They inserted something into the IV and when I woke up 20 minutes later, what was left of her was gone.

Usually, you eventually feel that all of the pain and feelings associated with a delivery were worth it. You bring a baby home and weave them into your life and that of your family. In my case, I had come to the hospital knowing I would be leaving empty handed. What I didn't appreciate was how that would feel in the ensuing weeks and months. I didn't understand how the weight of something like this could be borne by one person alone. How the gravity of this kind of situation could lie flat across your chest and stay there, perpetually, making sure it hurts to breathe.

During the two days I was in the hospital, I wondered how, exactly, the nurses and doctors could do *this* job. And only this job. Helping women to deliver dead babies all day, every day. I thought that you must have to check your soul at the door when you arrive. And that they must give it back to you when your shift ends, so you can go home and be real again.

In what would prove to be the hardest moment, by far, they brought her to my room. I had finally managed to dress myself. I was in tremendous physical pain, and no matter where I looked, searched, there was no baby to bring home, though I had felt her arrival. They had asked me a few times if I wanted to see her. They told me it would be good for me. They warned me that she was discoloured because she had been gone for quite some time before she made her way out and into this world.

A gentle nurse, a person whose face I have all but erased from my mind now, brought her to me in a basket, wrapped up in the tiniest white crochet dress and hat, wrapped further in hospital blankets. I hesitated, basket in lap, to pull the hospital blanket back enough to reveal her face. When I finally did, I saw that she was tiny, just a pound. But she looked just like him, and all the parts were there. Like a tiny doll, impossibly light, almost weightless. Eyes peacefully closed. Lips pursed. Gone.

For several minutes, maybe more — it's all a bit of a blur in so many ways and vivid in others now — I couldn't bring myself to touch her. Only to stare.

When they came to collect her, I realized I wasn't ready for them to take her away. They offered me more time with her, in another room.

They needed this delivery room for the next person who would endure what I just had.

That other room was like a living room: sentimental quotes about infant loss on the wall, footprints cast in clay, a Bible just in case. I sat on the leather sofa still clutching the basket. I shut the door to the room, which was inexplicably bright for such a shitty day. I unwrapped the blanket carefully and slipped my hand underneath her body, the emphasis on supporting her head, the only way I knew how to lift a newborn out of something, but she was weightless and I was completely thrown off. She fit, literally, in the palm of my hand, and my hand shook so vigorously at the surrealness that I had to put her down. I didn't touch her again, or see her again, after that.

The hospital told me that after 21 weeks' gestation, it's the responsibility of the family to "address the remains." Another jumble of words to say "bury her." I couldn't conceive of a scenario in which I'd be able to do this. I had never planned a funeral. Or arranged for a burial. I'd never done anything like this in my life, and the thought of doing it here, now, in this short window, was crippling.

I did the only thing that came to mind and I called my sons' father. While our differences were irreconcilable as married persons, we had the lifelong mutual objective of raising wonderful kids and always knew that it would take both of us to do it right. Our problem may have been that we'd developed into such a great team, playing logistical and schedule dominoes for so long, that we had forgotten about us. He knew where I was and what I was doing, as he'd held down the fort at home. And with only a few words sobbed out by me in a painkiller haze, he took care of it. Someone would come from the funeral home to take her from the hospital and everything else would be arranged. I didn't have to do anything. I had never been more grateful for him than I was in that moment.

When I got home, I felt like a lifetime had passed. Like a different mother had come home to my boys. I spent days, weeks, useless. Meandering. Sleeping. Waking from bad dreams and sleeping some more. I did little to take care of myself. I ignored the multiple calls from the cemetery and missed her funeral altogether. Days turned into nights without warning, and it was the nights that were the worst. It is still the nights that are the worst, the quietest, the loneliest.

In the weeks after, I came to feel a numbness. I thought that was my signal that I was somehow okay. That I had gotten over whatever there was to get over. There were kids to care for, lunches to pack. There was work to do here, paycheques to earn, chores to do, errands to run, and cats to feed. Some well-meaning friends had come over one night and hastily taken every single baby item in that tiny hall closet away. There were no more signs of her.

My real life, my real kids, involved lots to do, and yet I couldn't. There was some kind of hold on everything. Like I was standing still in the middle of an intersection while the whole world moved around me and I couldn't do anything to help myself.

Two weeks after Florence's birth, my first-ever nephew arrived. My sister underwent a 48-hour labour followed by an emergency Caesarean section to bring him here. I rushed to the hospital. It felt normal, and right. I was excited even. I drove 45 minutes, parked my car, took a ticket. I did all the normal things. And then, as if it was a symbol, I stepped over the threshold between parking lot and hospital and gasped. I was short of breath. And dizzy. Looking around, wondering what was happening.

It was panic. I wanted nothing more than to run a million miles away from there. Somehow I managed to make my way to her room, gift in hand, to welcome the most stunning baby boy I'd ever seen. I held him and choked back tears because he was so real. Heavy. Loud. Alive.

I thought of her. About how they would have been cousins, just three months apart. About how she was gone. Why she was gone.

And instead of being a remarkable time of solace, the advent of my new nephew blew a hole through my life. I wasn't as numb as I had thought. I wasn't over anything, not even a little bit.

There was no pivotal moment in the healing process when everything just clicked into place and felt right again. I wish I could say that I'm fine and that I never really think about it anymore. The truth is I think of her every day. Christmastime was particularly hard for me as I took my boys, as I always do, to see Santa and thought that there was something, a 3-month-old baby girl decked out in a ridiculous dress, missing from the photo.

Things don't get better all at once. They do get better, but I think, in many ways, I can never be the same person I was before I met her. I can never see a baby girl again without thinking of her. I can never walk by the hospital where both, all three, of my babies were born, without feeling grief, loss. I can never open the white lace-embroidered envelope that the hospital gave me when I was discharged and look at the photos of her and copies of her smudged footprints and handprints and all of her stats — time of birth, date of birth, date of death, birth weight, length, and name — without a rush of feelings inundating me, ruining the rest of my day.

It would take me nearly seven months to the day to finally visit her gravesite. I had tried, on so many occasions, to will myself to drive there. Half an hour away from my home, I knew, there was a Jewish cemetery where my Gentile baby girl was buried. I didn't know where or how to find her; I just had a set of coordinates.

A friend, a wonderful and patient soul, offered to go with me. So we drove together, parked at the side of the road, and walked up and down the aisles of graves of other babies. Sites where so many families must have come to grieve their own losses. Some had frozen-over flower beds. Some had stones with the babies' names, birth dates, pictures of trains or teddy bears. Some had stuffed animals, candles. And some, like the grave belonging to my little girl, had nothing but a stake in the ground with a paper card inside that said the family name. It had taken me so long to get here that the paper card was missing altogether, likely blown away in a past rainstorm. I knew it was her only by chronological order and location.

I had no idea what to do, or how I was supposed to feel, once I got there. In that moment, I felt lucky my two boys were waiting for me at home and that I hadn't come here alone.

It was the very last day of November and with it came cold and wind. I was underdressed for the weather and walked around so long my hands froze before we found her. I stood there, for what felt like forever, and took note of the size of the grave itself; tiny, just like her. I took in the dozens of other newborns surrounding her gravesite and finally started to cry. I cried because I felt some kind of shame, like I was less of a mother, for having left her here so long alone. For not having the strength to come here before today.

The rest of my time by her gravesite is foggy. I was sad, and relieved, but mostly sad. I left with the resolve that I'd be back again soon. And that I'd get her a proper gravestone. It was the least I could do to honour her little life.

I'm no longer convinced that time heals everything. Not all wounds, anyway. I think time gives us the ability to expand, to romanticize, to compare. It gives us time to grieve, and it is in grieving that we do the hardest work. It is under the veil of grief that we feel we can hide from the world, feeling sad and alone, desperate, and cursed.

I am convinced that the only truth about loss is that there is no truth about loss; all losses are experienced differently, taken on the chin or on the shoulders, or both. Each loss carries with it its own timetable, often independent of yours; when you wish to move on matters not, for the grief will dictate when you actually can.

I felt myself forget her just for a moment the other day, like something leaving my conscience. Not unlike those moments when you go from one floor of your house to another in search of something and forget what it was that you were looking for, but you know, without a doubt, it was something. It felt strange. And I guess the fact that I noticed it at all meant I wasn't really forgetting her. The strange and unexpected emptiness that had fallen into my lap all those months ago, the weightlessness in my arms, just changed ever so slightly. It was a relief, because for emptiness, it was so heavy to carry around.

When I thought there was a chance I could ever forget her, I cried. I wondered if ever there would come a day when I could actually do that, and it made me feel a million different ways. And then I took each of my sons by a hand, taking the spot in between them that would have undoubtedly been hers, and together we walked to the park: me flanked by two with one in my heart forever.

20

MISCARRIAGE AIN'T EASY...
BUT IT'S EASIER WITH
MORE THAN ONE PARTNER
BY YOUR SIDE

Jenny Yuen

WE EXPECTED A PICTURE of our little bean, something we could put on our fridge when we got home from the ultrasound clinic. At an estimated 12 weeks pregnant, this was our first scan. We were both 34 at the time. Weeks before, the Clearblue Easy test had flashed *Pregnant*, like I had won a prize on *The Price Is Right*. I actually breathed a sigh of relief. We had beaten the odds by getting pregnant before 35, when everything starts to go downhill. So the stats say.

What I've learned since is that a hundred — or is it a million? — things can go wrong between trying to conceive and a positive result. And even if you get a positive result, you're not out of the woods yet.

Miscarriage is nothing extraordinary, yet it certainly feels that way when you are going through it.

⌒

But my situation was indeed unique: I'm polyamorous, with two men as my life partners. There was Charlie, the father-to-be, and Adam, who is 30 years my senior.

Polyamory means being in more than one romantic, committed relationship at a time with everyone's consent, with a foundation built on honesty, transparency, trust, respect, and open communication. And, of course, love. In our structure, we are a "V," meaning my partners are not romantically involved with each other and I am the "hinge" in the middle.

The funny thing is, the three of us were in a love triangle for the longest time, and one of the big issues in deciding consensual nonmonogamy was my desire for a child. Adam and I had wrestled with the pros and cons: He felt he was too old; I wasn't sure, either. He already had a child from a previous marriage, who was grown. He didn't want to do it again. I wasn't sure it was fair for a child to have a dad so advanced in his years. And then there were all the health risks associated with mature sperm, including chromosome deficiencies.

Charlie wanted to see where a relationship would go with me. We met while he was in Canada to attend his father's second wedding. As fate would have it, we crossed paths in a Montreal chess café. He had to fly back to London a day after our first date in Toronto, and so it was hard to gauge if we had a future together, as we were only in the early stages of "dating" and there was an ocean between us. However, the more we saw each other — back and forth from Toronto to London — the more we discussed serious things: kids, family, marriage, all the checkpoints in the relationship escalator.

In 2015 Adam proposed the concept of trying to see if the three of us could operate as two separate relationships, but one where we'd work together: the V. They both knew about each other, but before we had the discussion about polyamory, I had always been told to choose one or the other. I didn't consider that there was another way. None of us did.

Charlie made the brave decision to move to Canada from the United Kingdom, and about a year later, we started trying to make a baby, with Adam's emotional support. They are metamours to one another — that is, the partner of their partner (me). But they've come to call each other "Co," as in *co-partners*.

⁂

The ultrasound technician rudely told Charlie and me to immediately go see our midwife. "You have to go to your midwife. I can't answer anything. Go now."

Having never been pregnant before, we thought it odd, but didn't know any better. We arrived at our midwives' office in Toronto's Regent

Park, only to be told the paperwork hadn't come through and that, normally, ultrasound technicians don't tell patients to rush in. We waited an hour before Jodi, our midwife, came in to look at our file.

She led us into her office and gave us the bad news. Even though we were twelve weeks in, our baby had died four weeks earlier, at eight weeks. She had just stopped growing. I'm not even sure it was a she, as it was too early to tell, but it felt like a girl to us. And a Chinese acupuncturist had told us that it was, so we went with that.

We were completely blindsided by the diagnosis. I asked for a second opinion. I hadn't had the usual miscarriage-type symptoms — spotting, cramping, bleeding. There hadn't been any indication there was something wrong. There still wasn't. My pregnancy symptoms had begun to taper off at nine weeks, but I read that was totally normal on a few pregnancy forums. Normal is different for everyone.

My hair was still thick from the hCG pregnancy hormones that pumped through my blood and my belly was hard and starting to protrude.

"We call it a 'missed miscarriage,' when the body doesn't clue in that the baby has stopped growing," Jodi explained.

Charlie and I had felt we were in the safe zone — at least the safe-ish zone — and had started to tell a few people about our baby bump. We left the midwives' office completely shell-shocked.

They say miscarriage isn't so much grief for the present as grief for the future.

I had pictured our future with *her* many times.

When Charlie was in London, he had told me about a dream he had about picking up our little girl from school, with a stop-off to the dry cleaners. He saw her, half Chinese, with little pigtails.

For me, I pictured him carrying her as I walked toward them down the aisle at our wedding. She would have been two months old.

At work, I was worried about getting laid off, and I wanted to see if I could take an early maternity leave. In fact, I had a meeting with Human Resources, which I couldn't bring myself to cancel, scheduled right after the ultrasound. I drove us home, trying not to lose it while on the road.

I thought about so many things: the stroller we had planned to buy at a Black Friday sale, the change table, decorating her nursery. Our midwives. I was looking forward to regular check-ups and delivering at Sunnybrook with them by my side. I couldn't wait to figure out how to breastfeed, clumsy and petrified, for the first time. We were going to tell our close friends in person later that month, on my birthday. I had even survived covering a story for the paper I work for about a nauseating poutine-eating contest when all smells — let alone visuals — made me want to hurl.

All these life plans stopped. Just like that.

It sounds cliché, but she felt like our tiny miracle, conceived on the third try. We had beaten the odds of conceiving before everything shifted into the high-risk pregnancy zone of 35 or older. The timing would have been perfect. But that's what you get with parenthood and life, I guess. Plans change and a lot of things are not in your control.

Growing up in a turbulent household, I was always unsure if I would be good with kids. Even during interviews with children, I found myself to be awkward. I never knew how to talk to them. I was uncertain about my maternal instincts and skills. But as my brief pregnancy progressed — dealing with round-the-clock nausea, fatigue, and food aversions — and as I started to picture what it would be like to be a new mom, going on new adventures with Lily, as I'd imagined naming her, I became excited. I became attached. More than I could have ever imagined.

The pain of losing her so soon and abruptly was heartbreaking. We told our parents. Charlie's seemed more sympathetic than mine, but maybe from Chinese parents this was their way of showing care.

"You've got to get to the hospital and scrape it out," my dad instructed.

My mom kind of blamed it on me. Or maybe she was more concerned about the optics. "Why did you tell people? Next time, don't tell people until you're eight months pregnant."

She had lived through her own story of miscarriage before she had me. It sounded like she'd had a blighted ovum. There weren't many moments when she would get emotional. But her sternness gave way to sorrow when she would describe "the one between you and your brother." There is a 10-year age gap between my brother and me.

I wasn't expecting support from my parents, but Jesus, I thought they would have had more empathy — or sympathy — than they did.

A surprising thing that shone through during one of the darkest times of my life was how being in a polyamorous relationship helped me — helped us. Though, I'm not going to lie, it was sometimes complicated. I was upset at points while grieving because both my partners, being men, couldn't fathom what it felt like as a woman to lose a child. How could they? I wanted them to understand. I came around to see how different everyone's experiences were and how their grief varied in shades and intensities.

It was all part of the grieving. In times of trauma, I'm always one to be rational and make sure the logistics are taken care of. We opted for the misoprostol route — drugs that that you take vaginally, at home, to induce miscarriage. I took the first dose at 7:00 p.m. and proceeded to lie in bed with a hot water bottle while binge-watching *Black Mirror* on Netflix. My friend Maryam kept us company and brought us bubble tea, which was a really thoughtful gesture both Charlie and I appreciated. The cramps began at 11:00 p.m., shortly after she left. They became intense, and soon the blood and clots flowed. I was forewarned by a friend who had been through the process to be prepared for the sheer amount of blood. There was tons, more than I had ever before expelled or seen.

It was less traumatic than I predicted and surprisingly more cathartic. Around 2:30 a.m., the sac came out. We just knew. Without being too graphic, we decided what was right for us would be to wrap her in a onesie we had purchased for her that read "Home is Canada."

Holding her together, Charlie and I both broke down, wailing our pain into the night. This would be the only time we would get to hold our little girl. We buried her in a peace lily plant that we keep in our apartment. Is that morbid or beautiful? Maybe both? It seemed to be the most respectful move we could give our embryo.

The bleeding and cramping tapered off around 7:00 a.m. when I took the second dose, and I believed the worst of it is was over. There was a moment when I was mad at Adam for not being there, as the miscarriage happened at home. It would have been a shared experience for the three of us to grieve and form a stronger bond together.

A couple of days later, Adam asked, thoughtfully and sympathetically, "Did Charlie want me there? I thought it should be a private moment for the two of you."

I hadn't considered that. So I asked Charlie and he said, "I think I was glad it was just us, privately."

It made me take a step back to recognize that in polyamory, you can still have private moments with each partner without the other partner(s) feeling left out.

As I recovered, I no longer felt pregnant, and depression set in. Week after week, nurses drew my blood to check my hCG levels. They weren't going down, indicating there was still tissue stuck in me. Pissed off, I realized we needed a night away to distract us. I took Charlie to his first-ever Medieval Times Dinner and Tournament to watch actors dressed up as armoured knights duke it out in a sandy pit on horseback. The same night, we came home and he inserted two more doses of misoprostol in my vagina.

I stayed up most of the night, expecting the same Bates Motel horror scene, but nothing happened. Not a speck of blood.

The next morning, Charlie had to go to work. I thumbed the online listings for an abortion clinic that was open on weekends. I found one and Adam took me. The dilation and curettage procedure was fairly quick but traumatizing. Following the procedure, as I sat in a La-Z-Boy recliner with other younger women around — women who didn't want to be pregnant — I felt like I was the only one in the room who was crying because I wanted to be. During the weeks that followed, I felt my best defence against spiralling down to madness was to seek out bereavement groups and forums in person and online. I stopped watching episodes of *Black Mirror* and instead watched Ali Wong's comedy special where she talked about getting her "miscarriage bike"; it made me feel better.

As a journalist, I have never been afraid of being open about my experiences. I posted much of my miscarriage experience on Facebook. I was surprised to be met with a flurry of private messages from friends — men and women — who admitted they had gone through losses of their own. Talking about my experience was what reconnected me to some friends I had lost touch with across the globe, friends who are undergoing in vitro fertilization or contemplating freezing their eggs or have been told they're candidates for early menopause.

I found reassurance and validation in their stories. They were not ashamed. Many didn't advertise their experiences when it happened to them, either. I felt the burden of sadness become lighter knowing that sharing openly helped them.

Meanwhile, Charlie was still processing his grief and so I asked Adam if he could take me to a Pregnancy Awareness and Infant Loss (PAIL) meeting. I thought connecting with a support group would be a good thing.

Fourteen of us sat around a rectangular table in a rented church hall. Adam listened to women talk about their stillborns and miscarriages. He felt compelled to speak about his own mother's miscarriage all those years ago, and about how there was a hint of melancholy when she would speak about it.

And, surprising himself, he delved into how he hadn't been so supportive about his late wife's miscarriage, but he understood now, through supporting me, why miscarriage was so complex. Unexpectedly, he started crying. Accompanying me was a cathartic experience; as he said, his late wife had had a blighted ovum, but he hadn't been very present during what she had gone through.

In the grand scheme of things, Adam was close enough to feel sorrow for my and Charlie's loss but also removed enough to support us both. It was a surprising bonus of polyamory I hadn't thought of.

I was glad to have gone to a support session, but I ultimately allowed myself to heal on my own terms and gave myself the time and space I needed to feel like me again.

There were some rough patches. I listened to a podcast on CBC Radio about three stories of miscarriage. One of them came from Toronto mayor John Tory's staffer, Siri Agrell, who described a raw, heartbreaking detail of late-term miscarriage. I sat in my car, while pellets of rain poured outside, and refused to turn off the engine as I listened. In her segment, she talked about how a new dad said she had a bleak outlook on life because miscarriage had left her with an overpowering pessimism. I can relate to her on that level.

Even moving differently after my miscarriage was a challenge for me at first, but eventually, doing sit-ups at the Y didn't make me want to burst into tears. For a while there, being able to do the simple act of leveraging myself up off a yoga ball was truly upsetting, without my protruding belly and with the realization that it was gone for good. Now, I see the ability to do a sit-up as a positive, the way I see my miscarriage as a scar that is healing.

Charlie and I recently went through a second miscarriage. This time, it was an ectopic pregnancy after our first intrauterine insemination cycle in November. My blood test after the two-week wait was neither a zero for "not pregnant" nor a five for "pregnant," but a murky and inconclusive three. A few days later, I had what seemed to be a period, but as I took my temperature each morning, I noticed that it stayed high and I had unusual cramping.

What actually — thankfully — had saved my bacon this time around was the Kindara basal thermometer I'd been using for more than 14 cycles. If I hadn't noticed the consistent readings of 36.5 degrees Celsius and above, I would have carried on with my day and, quite possibly, my right tube would have burst.

The doctor asked me to come back, as my hCG was now at 100.

"Your embryo was dumb," explained my doctor in the most awesome way possible. "It went down a one-way street. Namely, your right tube."

Two shots of methotrexate to the sides and a painful weekend later — not to mention three weekly morning blood work sessions — I was back to zero and ready to start again.

Adam drove me to the fertility clinic every morning for a week to have my blood drawn leading up to the insemination procedure and then for the weeks after my second miscarriage was diagnosed.

My emotional experience this time around is certainly different. When you go through a second miscarriage, you almost feel like this ain't your first rodeo. You don't plan for 5 or 10 years down the road. You literally take it day by day. Or at least week by week. I felt resilient in the face of the ectopic pregnancy — no sadness; I just wanted to get it over with and get back on the horse.

And 52 days later, I'm back to beginning again. *We're* back to beginning. And it's actually fine. We have all learned something from the losses, and in that sense there have been some gains. We've learned that each of us can grieve and support each other in our own ways. Whether it's my holding Adam's hand as emotion overwhelms him while he tells his mom's story, or his driving me to the clinics, there's more love for me when depression and pessimism sets in. In Charlie's case, he has his Co to give him the respect and space he needs when it comes time to grieve.

Whatever the outcome at the end of every cycle, I know we'll have each other's backs.

21

THE DANDELION IN MY BELLY GARDEN

M.K. Shaw

I'M 43 YEARS OLD, sitting on a black leather recliner, squeezing Silly Putty in one hand and my best friend's hand in the other. I'm wearing my mouthguard, typically reserved for sleep, so I can safely clench my teeth without further wearing down my enamel. Someone has put *Grace and Frankie* on the TV to distract me, but I can still hear the buzzing of the instrument drilling ink into my body. The intense, burning pain that rages up my leg is like an electric shock. I remind myself over and over again how much I want this, have wanted this for years, and how beautiful it will be when it is done. I chose this artist carefully because she does gorgeous work and is efficient. I believe this will be emotionally healing, a salve for my broken heart. I know there will be a moment of release and catharsis.

I grit my teeth and count down my exhales, waiting for an anticipated moment of relief. When it comes, the pain lifts and I feel nearly intoxicated with the heady sensation — for what seems like 10 seconds. It is short-lived. The pain that erupts when the needle meets my flesh is unlike anything I've ever experienced. Dizziness washes over me. I rest my head back on the lounger and breathe deeply to try to distract myself, just as I did when I was in labour. It does not work. I hold out for as long as I can and then ask the artist for a break.

After a while, the breaks are almost as painful as the process itself. Because I have fibromyalgia, my pain radiates long after the stimulus has stopped. I'm wishing I took steps to numb my skin before going ahead with this. But I'm determined and I want to do this. I can handle pain. Mummy always said that things that are important don't come easily, and I believe this to be true. It certainly has been true for me.

I sit for 45 minutes that feel like 5 hours before we call it a day. Near the end, I'm unable to check out and let my mind wander. My body begins to object to the process and my leg tremors so thoroughly that the artist cannot continue. Meanwhile, my entire body shudders with grief and pain. I cannot control the shaking in my leg or the sobbing that cascades through my body. A flood of tears erupts from my eyes as I weep. We agree that I will come back on a later day to finish it. Even incomplete, it is exactly what I wanted.

My tattoo is a dandelion, blowing away in the wind with a trail of watercolour and dandelion seeds, accompanied by three blackbirds. The three blackbirds represent my three miscarriages, and the dandelion symbolizes letting go while still remembering. The inspiration comes from a line in a poem written by a participant at my first writing retreat in August 2016. As soon as I heard the words *dandelion in my belly garden*, I knew it was going to be the inspiration for my tattoo. For years I struggled to find an image that properly honoured my lost souls, and that was it.

My belly garden was not especially fertile. In fact, it was decidedly and frustratingly not so, at least the second time around. My husband and I had been married for several years, and people constantly asked us why we didn't have children yet. Everyone who knew me knew how much I loved kids, especially babies, and how much I had wanted to be a mom since I was a child myself. But technical difficulties in our marriage made it impossible to conceive the old-fashioned way. And with each pregnancy announcement and new addition to my extended family, I grew more and more depressed with the barren state of my womb.

I was open to the idea of adopting and researched the possibilities. In or around 2004, the easiest and quickest option was adopting a toddler girl from China. I knew several people who had successfully gone this route. While I was sad at the idea of missing out on pregnancy and newborn baby stuff, I mostly wanted to be a mom, so I was willing to go ahead with it. My husband was not. In any case, a year or two later,

China tightened up its policies on international adoptions, so we no longer qualified. My body mass index was too high and our gross family income too low.

Time carried on and I continued to be unhappy about my nonmaternal position in life. Three of my first cousins announced their pregnancies in short succession. My envy raged and my sadness heightened.

I finally brought up my fertility issues during a group therapy session, having been too ashamed to do so for several years. The psychotherapist who led the group commented in her typical caustic way, "I don't understand what the issue is. All you need is a way to get the sperm inside your uterus. Surely there must be a doctor who can do the procedure for you."

I went home and searched online for fertility clinics, called the one at the top of the list, which did not require a doctor's referral, and booked an appointment. In January 2007, I was inseminated.

After the obligatory torture of the two-week wait, I went back to the clinic for a pregnancy test. Later that day, I received a phone call from my nurse. She said, "You are a little bit pregnant."

I was cautiously excited, as was my nurse. My hCG hormone level was 14 and it should have been at least 25, but it wasn't 0. I was advised to come back in two days to see if my hCG had doubled, as it was supposed to. Two days later, my hCG had increased, but hadn't doubled. I went back to the clinic again two days after that. And then again. Each time there was an increase in hCG, but it wasn't doubling. Somewhere in between clinic visits, I attended a family gathering and thought it would be a brilliant time to tell my family I was pregnant. I thought if I told people, it would all turn out okay. Soon after, I was informed my pregnancy wasn't viable. My family did not know how to deal with my grief in the midst of their celebrations.

My husband and I went through another cycle of intrauterine insemination, or IUI, in March 2007. And hitting two for two, I again got pregnant. This time it stuck and resulted in the amazing human being who is my son.

However, the trauma of my son's birth lingers to this day. It scarred me, both literally and figuratively. The doctors claimed it was an emergency Caesarean, but there was no emergency about it. I remember how cold and alone I felt in the operating room. People were buzzing around as if I were not there. Only my midwife stood at my head and stroked my hair. As I slipped into unconsciousness, I looked up at her face and thought, *This is the last face I will ever see.*

I came back to life on December 22, 2007, in a brightly lit hospital room, surrounded by people. My midwife put my baby boy on my chest. I feared I would drop him, not knowing if my arms could move. Panic filled my heart as I wondered what was wrong with him, because I was alive and I believed we couldn't both be okay. But he looked perfect, absolutely perfect. His face in profile looked identical to the black-and-white image I had seen on the ultrasound just a few weeks before.

I didn't know how many hours he had been alive outside my body. I didn't know I had been intubated during surgery to keep me breathing, until I was asked to announce his name and no words would come from my throat. I also didn't know until later that day my mom had been waiting for me outside the operating room, that she heard the beeps and alarms, that it wasn't supposed to take so long for me to wake up.

I never heard anyone announce that I had a boy, that he weighed whatever he weighed, that he was born at whatever time. I didn't hear his first cry. I wasn't a part of his first snuggle or his first feeding. My only memories of his first hours were what I saw later through a video camera.

We were sent home three days later with the loss of those precious hours still acutely felt by me, coupled with the trauma of the repeated unwanted examinations and interventions. Blackness filled my soul as I sat up awake and alone in the middle of the night, hooked up to a breast pump while my baby and husband slept.

The blackness eventually washed away after those early days of motherhood, and we settled into our new life. Our days were filled with long walks, activities that both of us enjoyed, and a sense of ease I had never experienced before.

A couple of years later, we had a toddler and were ready to try for a second child. I confidently expected I would get knocked up easily again and declined the medications designed to produce more and bigger follicles. The fertility specialist informed me, "There is a big difference between thirty-three and thirty-six." We decided to try unmedicated IUI again. A cycle went something along these lines:

When my period arrived, I would call the clinic to inform the receptionist. Day 1 was considered the first day of a full bleed. On Day 2, I would go to the clinic before work with the other zombie-like women. We all had tired eyes with just enough hope to get us there. No one made eye contact with one another. Some women had men holding their hands. Most of us didn't.

As I walked through the door of the plush Yorkville office, I would sign in at the clipboard on the counter. A checkmark was put next to my name to indicate when my blood work was done and my name was crossed off for my ultrasound. The phlebotomist took many blood samples to test my hormone levels and see whether or not I was ovulating.

A nurse would put me in one of the waiting rooms, and I would undress from the waist down and cover myself with a paper blanket. I'd remove my Diva Cup and hope I wouldn't bleed on the floor as I waited.

After, I would be invited to a darkened ultrasound room. I'd lie on the examination table and slide my socked feet into the stirrups. A white, condom-clad wand covered in cold gel would be prodded into me, usually with the doctor looking away from me entirely, focusing instead on the images of my ovaries on the black-and-white screen. The first few times, the wand hurt. But after awhile, I grew numb to the whole experience. I also started wearing long skirts for my clinic visits so I didn't need to bother with the false modesty of a paper blanket.

The doctor moved the wand around and clicked the mouse to note specks on the screen, reading out numbers to the nurse, who marked them in my chart. I would not be included in the discussion unless I asked to be. I maintained my own notebook where I wrote down the numbers of how many follicles I had and what size they were. The doctor would then inform me when I needed to come back to the clinic for more testing or for the insemination itself.

Meanwhile, I would see my naturopath every few days for acupuncture treatments. I avoided caffeine and alcohol and anything else I believed would be unhealthy for a prospective fetus.

Once my follicles were ripe and ready, my husband would go to the clinic and leave his semen to be washed and prepared for the insemination. I would stay at home in bed, burning a moxa stick over my uterus, as instructed by my naturopath, to warm my womb and thereby make it more receptive to the insemination.

A couple of hours later, I'd return to the clinic. Sometimes my husband would be with me, sometimes not. Sometimes my son would be there, especially if the insemination occurred on the weekend. The doctor would show me/us the vial of sperm and I/we would verify the name on the label. A metal speculum would be pulled out. I'd remind the doctor I needed the long one because I have a tilted uterus. I knew there was a note to such effect in my chart, but they rarely read my chart, it seemed. Sometimes they would listen to me. But usually they made an awkward attempt with the too-short speculum and then commented, seemingly surprised, that I was right all along.

With a pinch of pain, the long needle would be inserted in my uterus and I would lie there for several minutes with my legs held up. Usually we would do the whole thing again the next day to better our chances, just in case the math was slightly off.

After three unsuccessful unmedicated IUI cycles, I routinely accepted the drugs that were offered to me in order to help better my chances of conceiving. In April 2009, during my first medicated cycle, I got pregnant. I had two full days of being happy before I received a call while in the washroom at work. My initial hCG number had been okay, but two days later, it had gone down when it was supposed to double. I knew I was going to lose this pregnancy. I cried silently in the washroom for a few moments before shoving down my sadness. This was on a Thursday. The following Monday, I lost my job because of government funding cutbacks. I was escorted out of the building with all of my belongings. When I got home, the bleeding started.

Thereafter, I had two more unsuccessful medicated cycles. My doctor suggested I undergo a diagnostic test that I had not taken this go-around, but had at the initial outset. The doctors had believed I didn't need to repeat the diagnostic tests because I had gotten pregnant so easily the first time around. Because of the new test, we learned that scar tissue, presumably from my Caesarean, blocked one of my Fallopian tubes, thus effectively reducing my chances of conceiving by half. This also meant that many of my previous IUI cycles were a waste of time.

With this new information, the doctors suggested upping my medication so I would produce more follicles. There was a chance of conceiving twins, which I was not thrilled about, but I would have done just about anything by this point. The only thing I ruled out was in vitro fertilization (IVF), because it cost $15,000 we didn't have. Ironically, if I were to add up how much money we spent on the IUI procedures and the drugs, I'm sure we ended up spending far more than that.

In late October 2010, I went through my last cycle of IUI, a few days after my Bubby died. Though she was 93 years old, her death was devastating to me, and I shut down in grief. On November 12, 2010, I went back to the clinic for a pregnancy test. I had taken the day off work for my birthday. We were on our way to Riverdale Farm when I got a call from my nurse. When I answered, she shouted, "Woohoo, you're pregnant!"

I was stunned and told her so. Her voice got subdued when I told her about the bleeding I'd had, which I assumed was my period. She said we would know more after the next round of blood work. My hCG was high for a first blood test, so she suggested I might have had twins and was losing one of them. Or I could be one of those women who bleed during pregnancy. Or … well, we weren't going to think about the other scenarios until we had more information.

The bleeding continued for two days, but my blood work came back strong. I was still nervous, so we did one more test two days later, and everything looked good. By then, the bleeding had stopped. I finally accepted I was pregnant. I booked my midwives, told my closest friends and family, and walked around with a secret little smile.

Shortly thereafter, I was driving to work when I felt a warm gush. Instantly, I knew something was wrong. My heart sank. When I got to work and saw the bright red blood on my underwear, I called my nurse. She told me to come in right away. I informed my assistant I had a medical emergency and had to leave. I drove to the clinic. The ultrasound showed the embryo was smaller than it should have been at that stage, but the doctor wanted to wait for the blood work to come back before saying anything definitive. I was sent home.

When my nurse called, I could tell from her tone of voice that the news wasn't good. "I'm sorry," she said. She told me to stop taking the progesterone and the pregnancy would end on its own. I informed my boss I was not feeling well and needed to work from home the next day. I was later chastised for working from home. When I informed my boss that I had done so because I was having a miscarriage, he didn't seem to think that was a good enough reason. The rest of the week, I took the bus to and from work so I could rest while cramps ravished my belly.

I didn't have it in me to try anymore after that.

The following year, in December 2011, I learned I have severe sleep apnea. So severe that the sleep doctor was shocked I had been able to carry my son to term, because the lack of oxygen should have suffocated him in utero. I wanted to get back to trying to have a baby once my apnea was under control, but by that point, my then-husband was no longer interested in a second child. We separated two years later and are now divorced.

After my separation, I considered returning to the clinic to try for another baby. But it was more complicated without a man in my life. First, I'd have to find a donor for the sperm. And second, did I really want to do this on my own? Upon much reflection, I decided that I did not. I enjoyed the life I was sharing with my son.

For years, I carried an ache on the left side of my belly reminding me of the babies I never got to meet. I attended many therapy sessions, went to sweat lodges, and took reiki treatments. I named each one of my babies, said goodbye, and watched them fly away. Still, they have always been with me in that ache on the left side of my belly. And it has never been an ache that I could discuss freely with anyone. I was expected to just "get over" the miscarriages, especially because they were early in each pregnancy.

This tattoo gave me permission to acknowledge they will always be a part of me. I no longer have an ache in my belly. When I think of them, I look down at the beautiful piece of artwork that is a now a permanent part of my body and I acknowledge their importance in my life. I talk about them freely, with strangers and with family members who never knew them. I feel at peace.

22
ROUND TWO

Ariel Ng Bourbonnais

I'M RELIEVED I DON'T MISS Dr. Singh's call. I've been dying to know if my über-low egg reserve is now extinct. It's been nearly two years since I've tested my AMH levels and I've mentally prepared myself to find out I have zero eggs left, at the tender middle age of 35.

What's AMH? I had no idea until it was too late for me. AMH stands for anti-Müllerian hormone, and it's easily measured by taking a blood sample. This test is not currently covered by the Ontario Health Insurance Plan (OHIP), but I think it should be because it's important for women to benchmark their fertility health. And this blood test is a simple and quick way to capture a snapshot. High AMH generally indicates a greater egg reserve and better-quality eggs. Low AMH indicates a smaller reserve and sometimes that the quality is degraded, too. I tell myself it's okay if my eggs are now rotten because I've already come to terms with my infertility after one miscarriage a few years back and many more years of struggling to conceive. I recently asked my doctor if I could pay for the AMH blood test again because it's worth $75 to give me peace of mind, which is why Dr. Singh is calling me today. When I see her name pop up on my phone, I pick up right away. As usual, she doesn't mince words.

"Ariel, the rest of your blood work is fine but we have your AMH results and you are at 2.9." She sounds excited for the first time in our entire history of fertility-related conversations.

My coffeeless brain tries to compute what she's saying. "2.9. How is this even possible?" My AMH was recorded at 0.78 a few years ago. I didn't think I could improve my egg reserve at all and especially not by that much. It's truly inconceivable, pun intended.

"I don't know, but it's a good thing. I know you said you and your husband were done trying, but I think you should go back to the fertility clinic. This at least warrants another conversation."

"I guess we could talk about it again. 2.9, are you sure?" I ask.

"That's what your results say. I'll send your referral to the fertility clinic today, and if you don't hear back from them within a few weeks, you call and let them know you're a former patient of theirs and need to set up a new appointment."

I'm glad she outlined the exact next steps I need to take, because I'm in a state of total shock. Hell, I think Dr. Singh is in shock, too. "Thank you for making my day," I simply say.

I hang up and immediately call my husband, Lawrence. He's not going to believe that I went from the 10th percentile of fertility to the 50th. I thought I had the eggs of a 45-year-old woman, but now I am back in my true age box. I'm skeptical. Something doesn't add up and I'm trying to figure out what it is. I wonder if this is a miracle because of my recent lifestyle changes. I stopped eating meat and started doing cardio a few months ago. Could a regular trampoline class and no-burger lifestyle get me knocked up, with the help of my husband, of course? I'm confused but happy. Then I start to wonder if the lab made an error and my AMH is really 0.29 instead of 2.9. This would be logical, would make sense, and would align with my previous diagnosis. A score of 2.9 is heavenly, unimaginable, *luxurious.*

Lawrence picks up. "What's up? I'm about to leave for work."

"Dr. Singh called and my AMH is 2.9, not 0.78."

"See, I told you. I knew you were okay." He sounds so relieved.

"I'm going to book us in to see the specialist, Dr. Adatia, again. Maybe we can do the government-funded IVF this time."

My husband and I paid for one round of IVF two years ago because we wanted to save the government funding, in case we decided to proceed with an egg donor. The egg donor IVF is more expensive than my round of low-stimulation IVF was. My eggs needed to be more gently drugged because the regular doses of medication would have killed them off. During our IVF cycle, we retrieved four measly eggs and only one acted like it was supposed to with the sperm. *One.* This hurt even more when my best friend went through the IVF process a few months after I did and was able to retrieve 18 eggs.

We implanted the only egg with potential and it failed. My husband and I thought we were being smart by saving the government funding, but it ended up being a dumb decision because we didn't go the egg donor route. We gave up all fertility treatments when the IVF didn't work with my own eggs, and that was the end of that.

Or so I thought.

"Amazing, Love. I'm so happy. I knew it!" He is so happy that it turns my hardened heart as soft as a peony petal. I want to at least try to have his baby again. The worst that can happen is that it doesn't work, and we've already come to terms with a no-kids lifestyle.

Or have we?

A few days later in a bathroom stall at work, my absolute *favourite* place to discover pregnancy, I find out that, in fact, I am pregnant. I had all the telltale signs that week. I had tender breasts, I was peeing every two minutes, and I was exhausted. I just didn't believe it was actually possible for me to get pregnant again, so I read the signs as extra PMS fun.

"We conceived naturally," I keep whispering to myself over and over again. This week is madness: first my AMH levels are practically in the normal range. Then I'm pregnant for the second time in my life without the intervention of a team of specialists. *Somebody stop me.*

When I tell Lawrence, he proudly says, "Cool, I knew it." And he really did. Lawrence always believed there was a chance I could get pregnant again, but I shut him down each and every time. I owe everyone who's ever told me that miracles happen a formal, written apology. The pessimist in me now has to believe in miracles, because this truly *is* a miracle. If I thought my AMH returning to normal levels for my age was good news, this is cake on top of cake on top of cake.

That evening, I have a dream I'm shovelling heavy snow and when I turn around, it's magically all melted away. This is what it feels like to be pregnant after giving up all hope of ever becoming a mother.

When I call my mom to tell her I'm pregnant, of course she's ecstatic. My mom has been there through the thick of it and she knows how hard it's been on me and Lawrence. She mentions that Halo is a really cool name, and I say it out loud and agree it's nice. After our conversation, I listen to Beyoncé's song "Halo" and cry. The lyrics are salt on my heart.

Oh, how all the baby-related feelings rush back to me. I put up huge walls after our IVF failed, and here I am pregnant, wall-less again. Our new addition has a fitting new nickname of Halo and I think it's perfect. Lawrence doesn't like the nickname "because Beyoncé is annoying," which makes me laugh.

Sometimes, I play a game with myself where the next song that comes up on shuffle carries a secret meaning that will be important to where I am in life. Usually, the next song ends up being something like "Wake Me Up Before You Go-Go" by Wham! and the game ends as quickly as it begins. And yes, I, too, question my choice in music. While I wait for my eight-week ultrasound, everything becomes overly saturated with symbolic meaning. I repeatedly see 11:11 and 9:09 on the clock, both lucky numbers for me. I see new meaning behind the words suggested by autocorrect, and when I get to the subway at the exact right time to catch a train, I'm delighted.

But when I visit my family in London, Ontario, I get stung by a wasp for the first time in my life. On the drive home, a monarch butterfly splatters on the windshield, and I'm sure both insect events are bad omens for my pregnancy. I've never seen a butterfly on the 401 ever, so I'm shaken when I see one right before it crashes into the glass.

It's always been easier for me to find negative symbols than to see the good ones. I know I need to stay positive because it's what I *should* do in order to have a healthy pregnancy. *No good baby can be built from pessimism,* I think. But my heart was ruined at my last eight-week ultrasound, so I'm hoping for the best while anticipating the same outcome as last time: no heartbeat followed by a dilation and curettage (D&C), followed by abortion medications.

Unfortunately, my newfound excitement is short-lived, just like my first pregnancy was. Even though no one has outwardly said anything negative to me yet, I know my ultrasound is not going well. First, I have a transvaginal ultrasound performed by a trainee under the watch of a senior technician. Then the more senior technician does the deed, and finally, when I think my vagina has had *just* about enough for one day, a doctor takes the driver's seat because she "has to see something for herself." As the doctor moves the wand over my belly, the machine makes noises like Mario collecting gold coins in *Super Mario Land*. It's disarming to hear such fun arcade sounds that will eventually indicate such real-life problems. I can't believe this is happening again, but I can. This isn't my first no-heartbeat-rodeo and I know this pregnancy isn't going to be viable. Gut feeling. But my doctor has to break the bad news to me, which means more waiting. When the doctor leaves the room, I try my best to glean more information from Tatiana, the more senior technician. I figure if I ask the right questions, she may just break.

Innocently, I ask, "So at this stage, shouldn't I see a heartbeat?"

"Too soon."

Man, she's cool as ice, this one. "But I thought at eight weeks you definitely see a heartbeat, no?"

"Sometimes yes, but in your case, it's too soon."

FINE, TATIANA.

When she, too, leaves the room to let me change into something less breezy, I frantically take pictures of what I see on the ultrasound machine screen, determined to interpret the results myself as soon as I get home. When I try to Google my "results," I'm unable to find answers. I only see other women's messages desperately seeking the same answers with no luck. I try another search, inputting the numbers and symbols as if I were trying to crack a bank code, but Google doesn't help no matter how many times I type in the numbers.

A few days later, Dr. Singh calls to tell me I need to have another ultrasound in a week. No further information is provided except that it's too early to interpret anything. I wait another seven full days, cursing Father Time each and every long minute. I have another ultrasound one week later and I wait again. I thought the waiting between fertility treatments and pregnancy-test days were hard. That was nothing compared to waiting to see if my pregnancy is viable or not.

THE ECLIPSE

A week and a few days later, Dr. Singh calls me during the eclipse. Everyone is running outside with their paper glasses as I wait for my mood to turn dark indoors. She tells me I have a blighted ovum and my embryo didn't properly develop. My nine-week ultrasound shows a gestational sac but not much else. My uterus is a black hole, a universe of nothingness. *My body is a place where souls come to die*, I think. An open container of Clamato lasts longer than my pregnancies. It's like my body is an ambitious new baker who gets all the right ingredients but fucks it all up in the kitchen.

I ask Dr. Singh if she thinks I'll ever be able to successfully carry a pregnancy to term, and she says, in all honesty, she doesn't know. Now that I've had two concurrent miscarriages, it seems like my body may not know what to do. I've been thinking the same thing, and I'm glad my doctor doesn't sugar-coat my situation for me. Dr. Singh faxes a prescription for 200-microgram apo-misoprostol to my pharmacy so I can get the abortion medication after work today.

A violence curdles my thoughts. It's like someone spit in my water bottle, and I'm angrier than I was when this happened in round one. Why do I have to go through *the exact same thing* again? I can't believe I have to take abortion medication to clear my body out *again*. That I have to tell my loved ones my body has failed me *again*, that yours truly sincerely sucks at making babies. Signed, Ariel Ng. I cry because I don't know what normal is anymore. I think about the beauty and horror of dividing cells and how everything can go perfectly right or so perfectly wrong.

As soon as I get off the phone with Dr. Singh, an excited co-worker runs into my office and tells me I need to go outside to look at the eclipse. I look down at my keyboard, afraid to make eye contact with her, as if she is, in fact, the eclipse itself. "I'm just dealing with some stuff right now and can't make it," I say.

She thinks I'm being lame. "Really? Come on, nobody is at their desk. Go outside, someone will lend you glasses. It's so cool."

"Thanks, I'll try to make it out soon," I lie. She leaves my office and I quietly shut the door behind her.

I'm dealing with my own eclipse right now; there's no way I can deal with the real one. My life is suddenly filled with hidden problems I don't want to deal with. I email my boss to let her know I'm leaving work early and pack up my stuff. I text Lawrence to let him know I was right about my gut feeling and it's going to be a long evening ahead. He's sad and I hate how I'm responsible for making him feel this way. I know he will find comfort in his work and in keeping busy. I will find comfort in getting the embryo out of me as soon as possible.

When I pick up the abortion medication, I read the instructions on the pill bottle and sigh loudly: *Instill 4 tablets into the vagina as directed.* It's going to be a fancy-fun night, I see.

I subway home and take our dogs out for a quick walk. Once we are all back inside, I shove the pills deep inside me, wash my face, and eat some cherry crisp I made the night before. I put on a giant pad and jogging pants and think about why, *of all the things to make*, I made cherry-fucking-crisp. I'm going to have an abortion while eating something that looks like one. Originally, I made the crisp for a good friend's birthday, but I had to back out of the party because of my ongoing uterus soap opera. I'm tired of making excuses for my body's bad behaviour. I want to have fun and live my life, not sit at home waiting for the faux-life inside me to exit.

I scroll through Netflix and decide *Old School* will be my miscarriage movie this evening. I've been watching nothing but idiotic comedies because they're all I can stomach. I'm thankful I don't have to wait yet another week, finding gratitude in the little things. Even though I knew in my heart that this pregnancy wasn't viable, I still second-guess myself. It's hard not to. Maybe I shouldn't have dyed my hair just yet, or shared that entire bottle of wine with Lawrence. It's a strange feeling knowing you are carrying around a dead, or in my case, an underdeveloped embryo inside of you. I say to myself over and over that it's just bad luck, but I don't really believe it 100 percent. On some level, I wonder if I deserve this for things I've done in the past. I try not go there, but my mind often wanders to the shittier parts of me.

I search Google for the medication name and read that I should start to bleed between two and five hours from now. For a long time, nothing happens except I get extremely cold followed immediately by hot flashes, then chills again. I eat some chips and stew in despair. Lawrence comes home in a relatively good mood, and I immediately sour it with my angry emotions, filling the house like a diffuser. He doesn't take it personally, though — he's used to my infertility-related mood swings. He doesn't stoop down to my anger level, and I'm thankful to have a partner who is more stable in all things baby.

Finally, six hours after I take the medication, unbearable cramps start. This is way worse than anything I've felt previously. I ask Lawrence to get me three Advil. He tells me three extra-strength Advil is too many, but I strongly encourage him to comply. Somehow, he is able to understand my request through my clenched teeth and squinted eyes and gets me my meds. I can't believe I wasn't given pain medication along with the abortion medication. I hate that I am suffering on top of the suffering. I writhe, fever, and chill for an hour before the blood finally comes.

The blood is like heroin at this point — I can't get enough. *Give me more. Give it all to me. I want everything out of me NOW.* I should be more careful what I wish for because everything literally does come out. I wasn't expecting diarrhea along with the blood, but I am cleaned out in every which way possible. And when I think there can't be anything left inside of me, there is. I spend a couple of hours making my way from the bed to the toilet and back again. I think this must be the worst night of my life in terms of physical pain. I have a fever of 38 degrees Celsius and I wonder how long this can actually last. I'm in this alone because Lawrence is sleeping soundly; the man can sleep through anything. He has to work in the morning, so I'm glad he can get some rest as I dissolve my body and our little soul down the toilet.

When I wake up, I'm thankful the bleeding has finally slowed down. I'm going to be okay again. Eventually. *Physically, at least.* Lawrence comforts me the best he can and I accept it the best I can. It's all either of us can do in order to survive another big blip in our relationship.

I'm angry and I'm going to let this anger out whether it makes me feel better in the end or not. I've happily been a pescatarian for nearly a year, but after my medication evening, I go on a meat binge, eating all my favourite things I normally wouldn't ever touch: chicken fingers, poutine, Caesar salad with bacon, pepperoni pizza, and a Big Mac combo to round things out. I fall off the workout train and take comfort in cupcakes, candy, and chips. I'm too lazy to pull apart licorice, so I eat the intertwined strands as one. I dye my hair the colour of anger and cut it shorter. I wear black, not because it's the colour of mourning, but because it makes me look tough and contrasts with my red hair nicely. Maybe if I look rough on the exterior, my interior will toughen up a little, too.

The miscarriage decides to remind me it's still around for the next eight weeks. In turn, I decide to remind Lawrence every single day that I'm still bleeding. My miscarriage successfully ruins not one, but two closely spaced vacations, carefully saved for and planned for the end of summer. Nothing says vacation like wearing a thick pad in your bathing suit!

I decide therapy will be my shtick for the next few months. It should be more fun than going out for dinners and generally having a good time with my family and friends. I ask a trusted friend for a recommendation and set up my first appointment with Dr. Nyuli.

When I first meet Dr. Nyuli, I immediately trust and like her. She also has red hair, and I feel comfortable baring my most uncomfortable thoughts with her. She doesn't judge me and she tries to help me see myself outside of my overflowing feelings. This is the first time I've opened up to someone about absolutely everything. All the parts of me I hate are on display, and I feel vulnerable, scared, but also relieved I have an outsider to talk to.

However, weeks later, I don't know if therapy is helping or hindering. I find myself walking around saying, "I'm just the glass; the anger is the water. I'm but a container; I'm not my anger," as my face reddens in rage. Even though I repeat similar mantras to myself over and over, I'm not sure I really believe them just yet. I feel so sorry for the sperm who swim inside me, the poor little guys have no idea what they are up against. Trying to have a baby has turned out to be like peeling a hard-boiled egg. I thought it was going to be an easy task, a one-crack-and-peel kinda deal. Instead, I'm peeling tiny little bits of shell off an hour later, never getting to what I wanted in the first place. I wish there were a pill I could swallow to take away the angry. I'm not sad or depressed — I'm pissed beyond reason. People often say that attitude is everything, which angers me even more. Before my fertility treatment ended, I had my hopes up for a few years. To be let down again is hard on the soul. On the mind. On the body. On the relationship. On my heart.

Lawrence and I attend a neighbour's party, where we find out our neighbour, the one with the super-adorable two-and-a-half-year-old, is pregnant *again*. Her husband, who plays basketball with Lawrence, lets it slip that another one of our mutual friends is pregnant with their second child, too. I stand there trying my best to stay chipper, but I quickly feel uncomfortable in my hormonal acne and non-baby body. I hate how I can be in a stable mood and it can suddenly shatter into pieces all around me because of other people's happiness. I want to cry now. I'm thankful there are a few other non-baby ladies at the party tonight. I don't know them well enough to know why they don't have children, and I don't care to know either. It's nice enough not to feel alone for a few minutes before I ask Lawrence if we can leave the party early.

Although the physical experience of my round-two miscarriage lasts painfully long, it is much easier on my mind than the first one. I knew what to expect this time and mentally I did all the right things to help me heal. Or what I think were the right things, anyway. Besides therapy and indulging in a meat week, I let myself get away with other so-called bad behaviours for a limited time. I buy myself things I don't need and waste money on hair dye to make it more vibrant than it needs to be. I eat like no one is watching, I drink like Captain Jack Sparrow, and I almost enjoy every mindless minute of it. Life sure is easier when you're not really dealing with it.

My friend asks me if I am okay and I monotone-autorespond that yes, I am. But it's hard to break past the standard response. I'm not really sure what I'm supposed to say. I'm not really sure if I'll ever be fine with my situation, but I know I'll learn to accept it more every single day.

I guess the question for me and my husband is, Now what? We're at an impasse. I was so happy when we made the decision last year to give up on our biological baby dreams. It was a relief to finally move on with our lives and get back to living. Now I feel stuck again.

Lawrence is able to move on more quickly than I am. As I stand in my little puddle of grief and anger, he's already jumped passed it. In one way, I realize how lucky I am because he's so easygoing about what I want to do in all of this. In another way, it's harder because the final decisions are mine to make. I'm hyper-aware of everyone around us changing while we remain stagnant: "He's changed so much since he's had a baby." "She's the love of my life."

We don't get such relief. Lawrence is a trooper, though, and doesn't hold on to anger like I do. I would do anything to get into his brain and walk around a little so I could figure out how he does it.

I think about going on birth control to reclaim some power over the situation. But that would be sealing the door in thick lead, and I don't think

I'm ready for that big a decision yet. When Lawrence and I have sex now, I'm always a bit nervous. I can't help but wonder whether I will or will not get pregnant. I'm scared either way. The same thoughts whirl around in my brain over and over, never finding resolution.

Now that I'm a full-time member of the Infertile Club, I need to learn to accept both the good and the bad feelings surrounding infertility. I will always wish that having a baby came naturally to me, and I'm green-eyed toward those who get pregnant, who never worry about having a miscarriage. I was once like that. Once. And it was one of the best feelings in the entire world. When I was younger, I loved playing the Game of Life. I always got excited when it was time to add blue or pink "children" to the tiny cars driving on the board. This was before the years of gender neutral everything and I was also much more innocent. I never imagined my car would remain childless; it wasn't ever a consideration. My real game of life is much different than I ever thought it would be. Like trying on an outfit and looking at myself in a mirror that has what I lovingly refer to as cellulite lighting. Not cool and *very* unexpected. But I may still buy the outfit anyway and feel better in my dress in another setting. Perspective is everything, as is good lighting.

Many people tell me that we can try again and we shouldn't give up hope because we're "still young." And it's true that we aren't really that old. It makes it harder for me to explain to others that I may be young but my eggs are old and pregnancy is probably not going to happen for us unless we get an egg donor. Others ask about adoption. I wonder if single people who want children and haven't found a partner to do so with yet are asked the question as often as we are. Of course we've thought of adoption, but it requires a completely different mindset. If we decide to adopt, we don't want it to be a consolation prize. We want to be all in, and we just aren't there yet. It's too raw and fresh to make such big decisions.

I'm also scared to test my AMH again because I don't know if I can cope with somewhat regular AMH levels and what that means for Lawrence and me. However, Dr. Singh thinks my AMH levels may have been elevated because I was pregnant at the time of testing.

There is a lot I don't know, but I do know there is a certain beauty that comes along with real acceptance of a situation. I'm not sure why I was chosen to experience this agony, twice, but I'm stronger than I've ever been before. I hate the words *blessed* and *lucky* and I don't think I'm either. I'm grateful to still have a husband who loves me despite all the drama and failure. I have family and friends who love me unconditionally. And cuddles from my two fur babies remind me that love comes in all shapes and sizes. I've found deep catharsis in sharing my story and in encouraging women to get their AMH tested earlier than I did.

After everything, I've found a peace, albeit a sadder one. Like the smell of my fingers after a cigarette, it's comforting and wrong wrapped all in one. I think I've maybe come to terms with being fecund-not; I always liked wine more than fresh grapes anyway.

A NOTE OF THANKS FROM THE 16 PERCENT

We are eternally grateful to Scott and the team at Dundurn for giving us this opportunity and for their willingness to see the immense value in sharing these voices. To the many supporters who reached out to share their stories on the16percent.ca: without you we wouldn't have been able to launch the platform that led to the inception of this book. To Danielle Lewis for generously helping us find a (brand) identity. And most importantly, to the writers who have contributed their stories to this collection. Your bravery, openness, and trust in us to bring your experiences to light is something we will be forever grateful for. This book is, ultimately, for you.

EDITOR BIOS AND
ACKNOWLEDGEMENTS

ALLISON MCDONALD ACE is a writer, editor, and communications manager. After experiencing a late-term miscarriage with her second pregnancy, she became an advocate for sharing stories of loss through writing to help others heal and know they aren't alone. Allison lives with her son and husband in Toronto.

ACKNOWLEDGEMENTS

First and foremost, I have to thank my mom for instilling in me the love of reading and writing and for the many nights she spent giving me spelling drills, which, incidentally, set me up to be not only a writer, but an editor, too. Because of you, I know what unconditional love is. To my dad, for instilling in me the grit and fortitude to never give up, and for being proud of all my accomplishments. To the earliest champion of my writing, my Papa, whose overblown sense of my talent gave me the courage to keep trying. And to my Granny, who loved me the best while she was here and I know has never stopped from the beyond.

To my sisters in all but DNA, Andrea, Gina, and Naomi — you believed in me as a writer long before I ever could; I love you more than you know. Andrea, your unwavering support of my writing, and of me, has kept me going when I would have otherwise given up. To Richie, who's early vision of me as a writer living in a house on a green hill is one I still intend to fulfill. To Dave, who tells me he's proud of me for even the smallest of feats. To Faye, who basically taught me everything I know about how to be a writer and editor, but most importantly, for your friendship. To Kim, for reading my work with gusto and for all the heart to hearts. To Nicole, without whom I would not have made it in publishing and whose laughter brightens up the gloomiest of days. To countless more friends and family who have cheered me on along the way; I'm so lucky that there is not enough space to list you all here. To my partners in The 16 Percent, Caroline and Ariel, thank you for asking me to be a part of this and for showing me what women can do in the toughest of times.

To my husband, Eugene, an angel on earth if ever there was one, who has held me up when the burden was almost certainly too much, but never let on that it was: I love you deeply. To James, who gave me the gift of being his mother and for hugs that melt the whole world away: I love you through and through. And finally, to my baby girl, whose name is etched on my heart and who set me on this path: I am forever grateful that, in your place, you gave me a purpose to go on.

ARIEL NG BOURBONNAIS was diagnosed with premature ovarian aging at the age of 33. She found strength and resolve in knowing that sharing her experience helps others. She works for the University of Toronto and is in the process of completing a memoir, based on her personal experience with infertility, through the University of Toronto's Creative Writing program. She is a proud Torontonian, wife, and (dog) mom.

ACKNOWLEDGEMENTS

I'm going to call out a few very special names here. To the rest of my friends and family, who have supported me through it all, I love you very much! I would write a personal thank you to each and every one of you if I could, but it would be longer than my essay and that just wouldn't be cool. Let's hug instead, shall we? To my husband, Lawrence Cary Ng, this book is dedicated to you. I was lost for a long time, still am some days, but we made it through the storm of infertility together. I love you. To Mama

Bo, My Rock. You are the most supportive person on the planet. Without your love, and our *many* venting sessions, I wouldn't be where I am today. Katie, I couldn't ask for a better Mamma. I was so sad when I found out I couldn't make you a grandmother. Instead of feeding into my shame, you turned it around and made me feel whole and good enough, as I am. Thank you from the bottom of my heart. Shaughnessy Bishop-Stall, you made me believe I am a writer — albeit one who writes in run-on sentences, but a writer nonetheless! I'm forever thankful for meeting you. To Allison and Caroline: When we worked together at Oxford, it never crossed my mind that the three of us would be on this journey together. You are the best teammates and are both wonder women in my eyes. *We made a book!*

Special shout-out to the following individuals: Rolland Bourbonnais, James Bourbonnais, Shirley Nyuli, Jen McNeely, Cynthia Cyr, Joanna Tejeda, Isabelle LaRose, Jill McClay, Kimberly Prachar, Lisa Ball, Chloe Chaitov, Alexandra Rosenfeld, Lisa Bevacqua, Caroline Tascon, Hillary Lane, Richard Woodbury, James Moyer, Lisa Cavion, Caitlin Bourbonnais, Suzanne Krupchyn, Amber Pachla, Joanne Denley, Rebecca Eckler, Emma Ingram, Sophie Lamoureux, Theresa Lemieux, Eva Barnes, Brandon Ng, and all the wonderful people I've met in my creative writing classes who helped me along the way.

CAROLINE STARR is a writer, editor, communications professional, and community advocate. After being diagnosed at 21 with polycystic ovarian syndrome and later suffering a miscarriage, Caroline became committed to building community surrounding infertility and miscarriage and openly discussing their impact on families. She lives with her son and partner in Toronto.

ACKNOWLEDGEMENTS

The first thanks goes out to my family, particularly my partner, Matt, who has been very patient with my heart and body over the years. I'd also like to thank my son, Charlie, who I jokingly call baby beluga, because in many ways, he is my white whale, and my second son, who, if all goes according to plan, will be joining us a few months before this volume publishes. Editing a book of infertility and pregnancy loss essays while newly pregnant wasn't where I intended to end up, and not something I'd recommend anyone take on, but it's really been a reminder that this is truly a process that is largely out of one's hands. I found some reassurance in those early uncertain weeks in these essays, knowing that no matter what the outcome of my first trimester, or subsequent months of pregnancy were, I wasn't alone, and had a robust community behind me.

The first unofficial infertility and pregnancy loss support community I joined was my first writing group, whose members had all been impacted in one way or another, so it's sort of fitting that this project has come full circle into a book. I'd like to thank Niva, Nicole, Lydia, Season, and Eilish for sharing so much with me over the past eight years or so, and for hearing me when I needed it. To my 16 Percent partners, Ariel and Allison, I'm so glad we connected again, even if I wish it were over something easier. There's no one else I could imagine taking this on with.

I'd also like to thank all the women who have trusted me with their pain over the years. It's been important, hearing you and hopefully providing you with some solidarity during dark times. I know so many of you have gone on to pay it forward to others, and seeing the changes we've all made together around bringing the conversation of loss and infertility to the forefront from a place of secrecy has been truly incredible.